MATRIX FOR MUSCLE GAIN

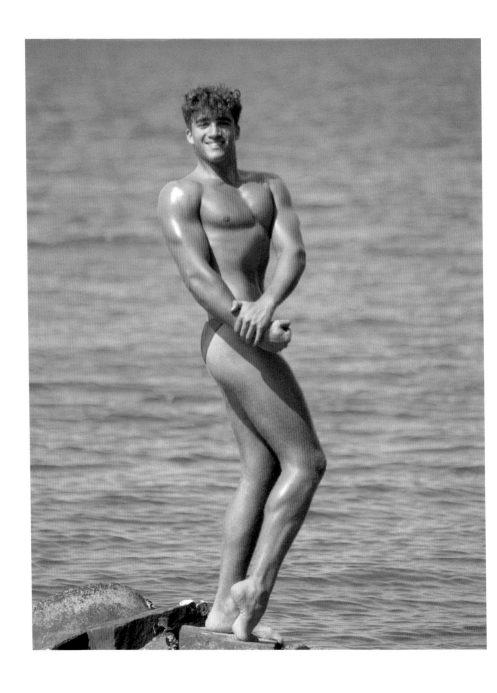

MATRIX FOR MUSCLE GAIN

Ronald S. Laura
Kenneth R. Dutton

ALLEN & UNWIN

To my son, Adam—aged 15—for having inspired me further to find new methods of building muscle without drugs, and for having used these methods to prove without doubt the remarkable results that can be achieved with Matrix training.

Ronald S. Laura

Title page: Adam Laura, aged 15, is proof of the success of Matrix drug-free training.
Back cover: Professors Laura (centre front) and Dutton (centre back) with Lin Mackie, Adam Laura, Gina Randall and Lee Priest.
Front and back cover photographs by David Adermann.

© R. S. Laura and K. R. Dutton, 1993

First published in 1993
Allen & Unwin Pty Ltd
9 Atchison Street, St Leonards, NSW 2065 Australia

National Library of Australia
Cataloguing-in-Publication entry:

Laura, R.S. (Ronald S.).
   Matrix for muscle gain.

   ISBN 1 86373 472 4.

   1. Weight training. 2. Bodybuilding. I. Dutton, K.R. (Kenneth Raymond), 1938– . II. Title

613.713

Set in 10½/12 pt Times by DOCUPRO, Sydney
Printed by South Wind Production Singapore Private Limited

The authors have great faith in this programme but cannot take responsibility for injury caused to readers. As with any exercise programme, it should be undertaken with care and with individuals working at their own pace. Seek your doctor's advice to ensure that you are in good health before embarking on this programme.

10   9   8   7   6   5   4   3   2

Contents

PART II: THE MATRIX SYSTEM IN PRACTICE

Acknowledgments

The authors wish to express their warmest appreciation to David Adermann for most of the photographs which appear in this book. Carl Hensel (pages 72, 123, 155), Kimberley Mann from Picture-This (pages 36, 97, 126, 130) and John Tirelli (page 182) are also thanked for their photographs. Sincere thanks are also due to Adam Laura, Lin Mackie, Tracey Moonen, Lee Priest, Gina Randall, Nerida Fittock, Leon Carlier, Tony Webber, Jamie Palmer, Peter Butler, Jamie Roberts and Steven Boland who appear in the photographs. Finally, we express our gratitude to Coral Johnston for the workout gear specially designed for this book. These and other items of exercise and leisure wear are available from the Corston-Mr Universe Collection, PO Box 39, Wickham, NSW 2293, Australia, Phone: (049) 50-2360, Fax: (049) 50-2360.

Preface

While the popularity of weight training in a variety of applications has increased dramatically over the last twenty years or so, it shows no signs of being merely a passing fad. The burgeoning 'fitness industry', the ever-increasing number of gymnasiums and the multimillion-copy sales of the leading bodybuilding magazines are ample evidence that the trend to resistance-based exercise is now well established — a counterweight, perhaps, to the increasingly sedentary lifestyle fostered by an affluent consumer society. Of equal importance in recent years has been the diversification in methods and applications of training, and in the types of 'consumer' making use of weight programmes. In sports training (for men and women alike), in rehabilitation after injury, and in general fitness programmes where weights take their place alongside aerobic regimes, the move has been in the direction of increasing sophistication and specificity of purpose; against this background *Matrix for Muscle Gain* evolved.

In our earlier work, *The Matrix Principle* (Allen & Unwin, 1991; 5th printing 1992), we introduced readers to an innovative approach to weight training which we have called the Matrix System. Our aim was to show how this type of relatively light-weight, high-intensity training could be used by a wide variety of trainers — old and young, beginners and advanced, male and female — to promote general fitness and overall physical development. In our book *Weight Training for Sports* (Transworld Publishers, 1992), we explored the specific potential of Matrix training as a means of increasing the strength and explosive power required for peak performance in a wide spectrum of sporting applications. In the present work, we focus exclusively on the use of Matrix routines to foster maximum muscle growth, and provide a more extensive discussion than hitherto of the theoretical principles underlying Matrix training. We also introduce a number of Matrix techniques not included in the earlier works, which restricted themselves to the twelve introductory techniques. Directed more intensively at increasing muscle mass, a further twelve techniques are published here for the first time in book form, and add to the variety. It is hoped that the final volume in the series, aimed at elite weight trainers, will appear in the near future: this will contain the final twelve advanced techniques.

Matrix for Muscle Gain is not a book for the raw beginner. The Matrix routines chosen for inclusion here are intense and demanding, as is the weekly training regime we propose. The specific purpose at which this book is directed — the achievement of maximum muscle growth — depends on this very intensity. Those who have not previously undertaken a serious programme of resistance exercise would be advised to complete the one-year programme set out in *The Matrix Principle* before attempting the more demanding routines set out here.

On the other hand, those who do have a background of at least a year's serious weight training — whether in Matrix or 'conventional' mode — should have little difficulty (given a short period of adaptation) in mastering the exercises shown in the following pages. Allowance has been made for those who cannot maintain the maximum rate of progress specified, and suggestions are given in the text as to how the programme may be spread over a longer period to take account of the trainer's individual capacity.

For those 'conventional' weight trainers and bodybuilders who have reached a plateau or sticking point in their training, and who cannot seem to increase their muscle mass no matter how hard they try, rest assured we are convinced by almost fifteen years of rigorous testing that a switch to the Matrix techniques set out here will be the most effective means of achieving the 'breakthrough' that has so far eluded them. In particular, we hope that those who may otherwise be tempted to resort to anabolic steroids and other harmful drugs in pursuit of muscle growth will join the ranks of the numerous Matrix trainers who, in our testing programme, have achieved equivalent results by means of this safe and wholly natural alternative. And for those who have completed the introductory course set out in *The Matrix Principle*, these more advanced routines will enable them to build further on the gains they have already achieved.

Introduction

Although it is only in recent years that Matrix weight-training routines have been widely published, the research and development that led to the evolution of the Matrix System go back to the late 1970s when the first routines were devised and trialled. Since that time, successive series of controlled trials involving hundreds of subjects have been conducted in both the USA and Australia. In each of the trials, groups of trainers carefully matched for age, sex, training level and degree of fitness were compared in terms of strength and muscle gain. A Matrix group and a control group (the latter undertaking conventional weight routines) each undertook a training regime of the same workout length and frequency, covering the same body parts, while all other variables (including diet, rest, and other forms of exercise) were maintained at comparable levels for the two groups. At the end of each trial period, the two groups were compared in terms of weight, critical measurements (shoulder girth, chest, waist, arms, thighs and calves) and strength levels.

Details of these clinical trials were provided in our earlier book *The Matrix Principle* (p. xii), but the results are worth reproducing here:

> On average, five out of six subjects in the Matrix groups showed gains in both size and strength significantly greater than in the conventional group. Some gains in size made by the Matrix groups at the completion of the course were as much as three times the gains made by the conventional group. Similarly, gains in strength by the Matrix group surpassed those of the control conventional group by a factor of 2 to 1. For every strength gain of five kilos made by the conventional groups, the Matrix groups exhibited gains of ten kilos.

In more recent years, the Matrix trials have in some cases been combined with controlled tests of dietary supplements, and the findings of these tests are reported later in this book (see 'Diet and supplementation').

Over the fourteen years since commencement of the trials, the opportunity has been taken to test various new Matrix routines, and combinations of routines, as these were devised. Some were rejected as less effective than others, while those which were retained were classified according to their usefulness in promoting aerobic efficiency, strength/power, and muscle size. In all, 36 Matrix techniques (twelve introductory, twelve intermediate and twelve advanced) have been thoroughly tested under clinical conditions. *Matrix for Muscle Gain* brings back the twelve basic Matrix techniques together with a further twelve techniques chosen on the basis of their effectiveness in fostering muscle growth; the 24 techniques are set out in combinations specifically designed to elicit the maximum muscular response.

All of the body-part workouts (i.e. combinations of routines) reproduced later in this book have been fully tested in controlled conditions by groups of trainers in the Matrix clinics conducted by Professor Ronald S. Laura, and have demonstrated their effectiveness in promoting muscle growth, even amongst trainers who already exhibited considerable muscle mass. There is a sequential order to the 24 techniques, in that each represents an increased level of difficulty and training intensity. This being so, the particular configuration of routines and the pattern of exercises therein are of paramount importance in maximising the growth-enhancing potential of Matrix training.

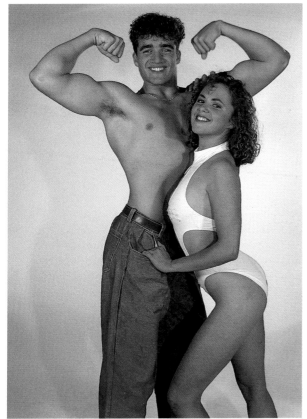

Adam Laura and Nerida Fittock, two young bodybuilders trained in the Matrix technique to great effect.

Chapters 1 to 3 set out in summary form the theoretical background against which the Matrix System has been devised and subsequently refined. Though some readers may wish to move straight to the exercises themselves, we hope that they will take the time to acquaint themselves with this earlier part of the book, which we see as fundamental to our approach to weight training in general — an approach which may be characterised as follows:

- *A pedagogical approach* We have tried to avoid the common tendency in weight-training instruction to rely simply on telling the learner what *to do*, without any indication of *why* he or she should do it. All too frequently, instructors — and even textbooks — simply prescribe a programme to be followed without indicating why or how it is meant to work. As professional educators, we are committed to the view that one's aim in learning is to become *self-directed* and, through understanding, to free oneself progressively of the need to follow blindly the instructions of others.

- *A holistic approach* We stress that weight training is most effective when it is part of a total fitness-oriented regime, which involves a number of lifestyle-related factors such as a healthy diet and the avoidance of harmful substances. In the area covered by the present work — the development of advanced muscularity — we are aware that many readers will be, at some time or another, tempted to resort to the use of artificial growth-enhancing drugs, notably anabolic steroids. An important part of our intention here is to present trainers with a *natural alternative* to steroids and other drugs which has proven itself more effective in this regard than any conventional training system with which it has been compared.

- *A scientific approach* Although there is still much to be learned about the processes and mechanisms leading to muscle growth, we believe that the only valid approach to more effective training lies in a better understanding of those processes. We do not believe in miracle methods of muscle gain, and are not presenting Matrix exercise as some mysterious or magic means of enhancing muscle mass. To some extent, it is true, the claims of Matrix training must rest on the results achieved, but it is important that any exercise theory which makes claim to effectiveness should also be able to stand the test of scientific analysis. While works on sports training have in recent years incorporated the most up-to-date findings in human physiology and sports science, it is fair to say that the majority of muscle-building manuals have been content to rely for their theoretical basis on bodybuilding 'folk-lore' rather than on advances in scientific knowledge.

Readers are referred to *The Matrix Principle* for a general discussion of the biomechanics of muscle action, the chemical and metabolic processes involved in the production of muscular energy, and the place of genetic determinants and ergogenic aids in individual capacity for muscle growth.

In the present volume, the introductory discussion will be restricted to the issue of muscle growth (or hypertrophy) which is the purpose for which the ensuing Matrix workouts have been designed. Our aim will be to examine, in the light of contemporary findings in exercise physiology, the variety of stimuli which combine to favour the maximum hypertrophic response in skeletal muscle. We shall see how Matrix training is designed to take the fullest advantage of these stimuli in order to promote fast and effective muscle growth.

Bodybuilding writers and competition judges often refer to an individual as displaying 'quality muscle'. This is a subjective term and is not easy to define with precision, but most advanced weight trainers will recognise the qualities to which it refers: the physique has a 'finished' look, the muscles well rounded and clearly defined, with good separation between muscle groups and a relative absence of subcutaneous fat so that individual bands or striations of muscle are fully visible and all major muscle groups are equally well developed. Trainers who are prepared to devote their time and energy to following the intensive intermediate Matrix routines will find them of invaluable assistance in promoting that degree of impressively visible muscularity which characterises the quality physique.

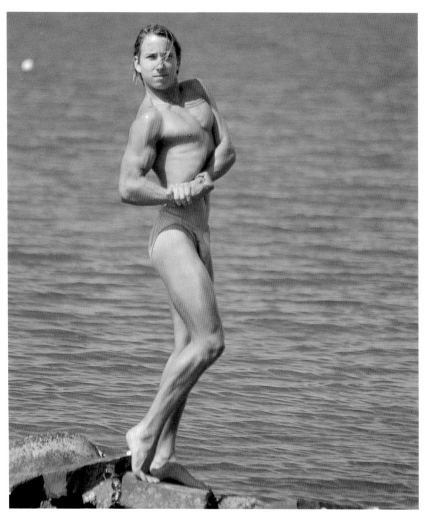

With a Matrix-built physique of great potential, 16-year-old Steve Boland has found inspiration from champion Matrix-trained bodybuilders Lee Priest and Gina Randall (opposite).

Part I

The Matrix
System approach

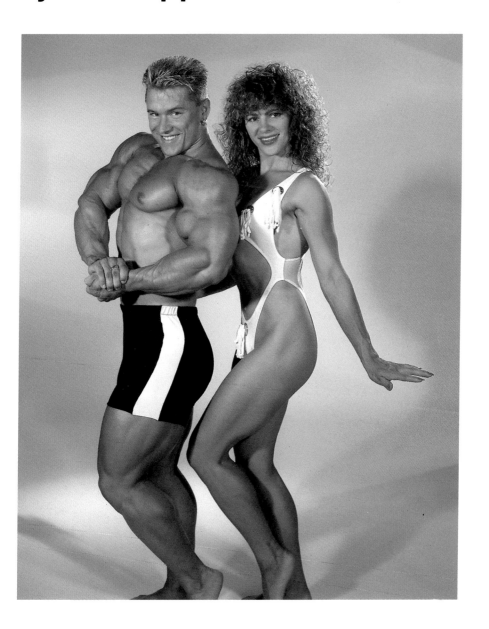

1   How muscle grows

Let us begin with a frank observation by one of the world's leading experts in the field of exercise physiology, Dr J.G. MacDougall of McMaster University, Canada. He has written that 'the mechanisms by which a program of near-maximal contractions results in enhanced protein synthesis and larger muscle fibers are not known'.[1] This statement, made in 1984, remains valid today. It may seem at first an astonishing admission, given the vast amount of scientific study that has been devoted to the human muscular system and the voluminous literature which exists on the chemistry and neurophysiology of skeletal muscle and its activity. Yet the fact is that much still remains to be discovered concerning the fundamental cause of the changes occurring in the muscular system in response to various patterns of exertion, and that competing (and at times conflicting) theories continue to emerge in the scientific literature and in discussion at international congresses.

This does not mean that we are in a state of ignorance as to the growth-response of muscle in relation to exercise. We do know what typically happens, and there is a considerable body of evidence linking various forms of muscular response to certain patterns of muscle fibre contraction. What is not clear is *why* particular patterns of muscle fibre excitation produce a greater growth-response than others. The evidence, in other words, is largely empirical; that is, it is based on the testing of alternative forms of muscle stimulation (usually through exercise, but also through mild electric stimulus) in a number of groups of subjects, and correlation of the results obtained in terms of measurable outcomes—which may include gains in endurance, power (strength x speed) or increase in whole-muscle size.

Exercise physiology is, by its very nature, an *applied* science, concerned with the practical application of knowledge in the field of human physiology generally to the performance of various exercise-related tasks, and for this reason the experimental data it typically uses relate to the comparative performance in specific activities of experimental and control subjects. By proceeding in this way, it can be demonstrated that particular forms of repeated muscle fibre stimulation are typically associated with particular forms of response, even if we are not entirely sure why it is that a causal relationship exists between them.

The Matrix System has been designed to take advantage of the most recent findings in exercise physiology relating to the patterns of muscular contraction which are closely correlated with an enhanced growth-response in muscle fibre. Some of the more significant of these findings are outlined in the following sections.

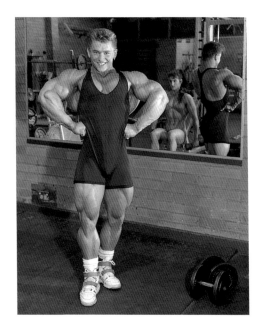

Lee Priest displays one of the world's best Lat spreads.

The stimulus

It is an elementary tenet of physiology that a muscle responds directly, not to a load, but to an electrical stimulus—a signal which activates receptors in the muscle fibre and causes it to contract. This stimulus is usually neuromuscular (i.e. transmitted from the brain by way of the motor nerve system), but it has been known since the eighteenth century that the signal may also be conveyed 'artificially' by means of a low-level electrical current transmitted by an electrode. This process was described in detail in *The Matrix Principle* (pp. 19–22).

Although artificial stimulation of muscle is able to mimic many of the effects of 'natural' (neuromuscular) excitation—it has been used in rehabilitative medicine and even in bodybuilding training—there is recent evidence to suggest that it does not fully replicate the effect of voluntary stimulation.[2] In terms of strength, for example, it has been shown that the intrinsic contractile force of a muscle (as measured by maximum twitch and tetanic tension evoked by electrical stimulation) may remain the same before and after a period of strength training, yet voluntary strength may increase markedly. Stated in less technical language, there may be a significant difference between 'evoked' strength (the strength of the muscle when contracted to its maximum by rapidly repeated artificial stimuli) and 'voluntary' strength (the strength of the muscle when contracted deliberately against the resistance of a weight or similar object). In tests based on longer periods of training, both evoked and voluntary strength increased, but the percentage increase in voluntary strength was twice the percentage increase in evoked contraction strength.[3] It seems clear, then, that the muscular strength that we can produce voluntarily or intentionally (by sending a message from the brain) involves factors additional to the purely physiological process of fibre stimulation.

In other experiments, it has been demonstrated that the initial gains in

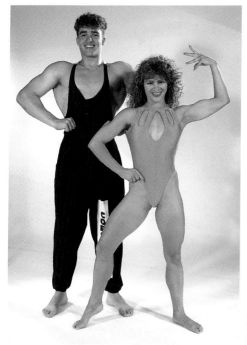

Adam Laura and Gina Randall exhibit the aesthetic benefits of Matrix training for fitness.

strength which take place during a training programme occur very rapidly—even in the course of the first training session—and that this cannot be accounted for by adaptations within the muscles themselves.[4] Obviously, the muscles have not had time to grow larger, and thus increase their inherent contractile power, within the short time-frame of a single training session. Something else—an 'extra-muscular' factor—must clearly be at work here.

Both these sets of experiments indicate that, even in the absence of adaptation (i.e. increase in strength) in the muscles, strength and power *performance* may increase, and it has been concluded that this is due to changes taking place, in response to training, within the central nervous system. This phenomenon is known as *neural adaptation*: strength and power training cause changes within the nervous system that allow a trainer to activate the muscles more fully or improve the coordination of voluntary contractions.

The power of extra-muscular factors to affect strength output has been confirmed in further studies. In one of these, when one limb of an individual was trained and the other (contralateral) limb was left untrained, voluntary strength per unit cross-sectional area (MVC/CSA) increased not only in the trained but also in the untrained limb; again suggesting that the change was due to neural adaptation rather than to qualitative changes in the muscles. In a separate study, trainers under hypnosis exhibited increases in voluntary strength: here, the least enhancement took place in the case of a trained weight-lifter, whereas the greatest effect was shown in a person who had always avoided physical exertion.[5] The conclusion, again, is that untrained people may have 'untapped' resources of functional strength which are normally inhibited by neural control mechanisms (probably in diffuse centres of the cerebral cortex).[6] These may be released when the inhibition is removed.

The implications of these studies are considerable, as they indicate the extent to which *learning* a muscle movement affects the force or strength with which we can perform it. Indeed, repeated research studies have shown that even experienced weight-lifters and strength trainers, when tested with exercise methods that are unfamiliar to them, do not have a higher MVC/CSA than untrained control subjects.[7] They are, of course, stronger in absolute terms, but that is because their muscles are larger; their ability to recruit their strength potential, however, may be no greater than in untrained subjects, because this ability is, at least to some extent, a learned response.

These findings underline the importance of neural adaptation in the effort required in order to exercise muscular force; we can say that when a given force is required to move a load, that force can be produced more easily by a subject who has learned the movement required than by one who has not. The neural adaptation that has taken place enables trained subjects to recruit their force potential more effectively, and thus to move a heavier weight without an increase in muscular effort. As D.G. Sale has put it, 'Strength and power training may cause changes within the nervous system that allow an individual to better coordinate the activation of muscle groups, thereby effecting a greater net force, even in the absence of adaptation within the muscles themselves'.[8]

The above experiments have generally related to the early weeks of weight training. What is the situation when training has been carried out for a longer period? There is evidence to suggest that, once initial neural adaptation has taken place, it is no longer called upon as a reserve to increase strength, as its place is taken by the growth in the muscles themselves.[9] To quote Sale again, 'As training is prolonged and muscle adaptation (hypertrophy) predominates, the decrease in specific tension may cause MVC/CSA to decrease toward the pretraining level'.[10]

The question thus arises whether it is possible to prolong the potentiating effect of neural adaptation beyond the early phases of training, so that the resulting increase in strength may be applied to maximising the hypertrophic effect of training. If, as seems likely, the initial neural adaptations act to trigger the subsequent hypertrophic response, it could be possible to maintain this triggering effect much longer into the training regime so that it does not cut out once the muscles themselves have adapted by growing larger.

If we consider the conventional weight-training regime, we can see how such a theory might apply. Let us take, for example, the biceps curl, and assume that a trainer does three sets of ten curls at each arm training session. As the trainer's strength increases and the biceps become larger and more powerful, the trainer can add more weight to the bar. This process will usually continue until a point is reached where the trainer can no longer keep adding weight and still perform three sets of ten. This becomes the trainer's sticking point.

Most trainers, however, will recognise that this point is not their absolute limit in strength, and will attempt to break through this barrier or plateau in their training. They may increase the weight and do fewer sets, or alternatively maintain the weight and do as many reps as possible of a fourth set. Generally, however, they will find that neither of these strategies is of assistance in breaking through the barrier when, in subsequent training, they again perform three sets with their previous maximum weight. The sticking point remains.

What has happened in the process of reaching this presumed maximum point of their capacity? Broadly, two things: first, their bicep muscles have grown stronger; assuming that the reps have been done strictly and the assistance of synergist muscles has been minimised, the biceps will have undergone a marked increase in strength since training began, as measured by the amount of weight they are now lifting. Second, trainers will have found that their biceps perform the movement more efficiently. If, for instance, instead of gradually progressing to their maximum weight they stayed with two-thirds of that weight and kept doing curls at that weight from week to week, not only would muscle growth cease at an earlier point but (as is common experience) they might even lose some of their earlier gains in muscle size. The weight (two-thirds of their maximum) which presented a challenge to the muscles when they first reached it, has now become easier to lift because of the muscular adaptations that have taken place, and the principle of conservation of energy has come into play.

The body will seek to expend the minimum amount of energy required for a given task. Particularly when this is a *learned* task, the amount of energy required tends to drop noticeably as the task is mastered and coordination improves. As the muscles can now lift the two-thirds maximum weight with greater efficiency than at first, the amount of muscular effort required drops accordingly; not only will no further growth be elicited from the muscles involved, but they may actually grow smaller as the task they are called on to perform becomes easier. This is not a problem confined only to novices: it is more likely to affect more advanced trainers, who have gone beyond the early period of rapid muscle growth and strength gain and are now regularly using quite heavy weights. Although doing the same amount of weight work from one week to the next, they either show no further gains in muscle or actually watch in frustration as their muscles grow smaller.

The problem remains that, even when exercising with maximum weight and at maximum efficiency, a plateau is still reached. Muscle fatigue sets in (at the end of, say, the third maximum set), even though the muscles are capable of more work. The usual answer to this problem is to take a few minutes recuperation, then to repeat the sets or to perform a number of sets of a slightly different exercise (say, incline dumbbell curls). Both these are effective methods of increasing the workout effect, as weight trainers have found for generations. Essentially, however, they merely repeat the effect of the first three sets: a maximum weight is reached, and thereafter there can be no further improvement. Once the body has fully learned the movement, there is no further challenge to the muscle system. No more weight can be piled onto the barbell or dumbbells, and any further challenge can result only from more and more sets at maximum capacity.

The Matrix System approaches this problem in a different way, by totally eliminating the concept of a 'standard' set. Instead of a set of say ten repetitions, all of them the same, which are performed at the maximum weight that can be lifted for say three sets and then followed, after a recuperation period, by three more sets of the same type, the Matrix set is made up of a pattern of *different* movements. Some are full repetitions, some half-repetitions (half-up or half-down), others (depending on the particular routine) may be one-third, three-fifths or some other fraction of a full repetition, while others again will be held isometrically for a period.

By this means, the response required of the muscles is constantly varied so that it is practically impossible for the neuromuscular system to learn a set. One helpful (if slightly inaccurate) way of describing this process is to say that the muscles cannot 'anticipate' what the next movement will be—it may be the same as the previous one, or a different movement—and in that sense we sometimes speak of Matrix training as based on the principle of 'muscle confusion'. A more exact term would perhaps be 'neural confusion', in that the neural adaptations, which are usually learned early in the training process and once learned play no further part in muscle training, are here constantly challenged into action and play a continuing part in the exercise regime.

Research by the eminent physiologist J.V. Basmajian confirms this hypothesis by using electromyography (the use of electrodes to measure muscular action potentials). 'The constant repetition of a specific motor skill', he writes, 'increases the probability of its correct recurrence by the learning and consolidation of an optimal anticipatory tension'.[11] Noting that the time required to train individual motor units is longer in trained than untrained subjects, Basmajian accepts the theory first postulated in 1964 that the acquisition of a new motor skill leads to the learning of a certain 'position memory' for it. He concludes:

> If anticipatory tensions and position memory, or both, are learned, spinal mechanisms may be acting temporarily to block the initial learning of a new skill. Perhaps some neuromuscular pathways acquire a habit of responding in certain ways and then that habit must be broken so that a new skill may be learned'.[12]

The question of how to overcome the effects of position memory in order to increase the impact of the training experience on the muscle system is thus of considerable importance.

In this respect, each Matrix set becomes a new learning process, and one that can never be fully mastered as each Matrix routine is different from each of the others. The neural input into contraction force is thus maintained at a level well in excess of that involved in conventional training, so that its potentiating effect on the muscles themselves is more fully utilised. While it is impossible to be entirely conclusive in this area, we can postulate that the rapid muscle growth which is usually observed after the first few weeks of training tapers off to a much slower rate thereafter due to the 'fall-off' in novel stimulus which occurs as repetitive movements are learned. On this basis, it could be concluded that the enhanced effectiveness of Matrix training is due in part to the constant variations in repetition which to some extent replicate the conditions of the early weeks of training, thus fostering the more rapid rate of muscle growth which is characteristic of this early period of adaptation.

Motor unit recruitment

A number of definitions are necessary at this point. Firstly, the 'motor unit'. Each muscle fibre is, we have seen, activated by a nerve fibre which conveys the message from the central nervous system which 'tells' a muscle to contract. But there is not a one-to-one relationship between nerve fibre and muscle fibre; if it were so, there would need to be enormous numbers of nerve fibres, each connected to a single muscle fibre, and the nerve trunks would need to be very thick indeed. Rather, each nerve fibre activates a group of muscle fibres, consisting of as low as five fibres in muscles controlling fine movements (e.g. the human extraocular muscles) and up to 2000 fibres in large coarse-acting muscles (e.g. the medial head of the gastrocnemius): these groupings are known as *motor units*.[13] The muscle fibres which make up a motor unit are not grouped together, but are scattered about the body of the muscle and intermingled with fibres of other units.

Secondly, we need to understand the notion of 'recruitment'. Like the concept of the motor unit, this was first developed by the pioneering neurophysiologists Sherrington and Adrian in the 1920s, and is now recognised by motor systems physiologists as the primary mechanism for the control of muscle force. It proposes, in simplified terms, that the tension developed by a muscle depends on the addition (or *recruitment*) of more and more active motor units. In general, these units are progressively recruited (under increasing tension) in an orderly sequence, those with a low threshold being recruited first, those with higher thresholds later: this is known as the concept of threshold grades, according to which the motoneurons innervating a muscle can be scaled according to relative intensities of synaptic input (i.e. input at the nerve-to-muscle junction or synapse).

In progressive muscle contraction, two things occur: more and more motor units are activated or 'fired', and the rate of firing progressively increases. The order of firing (or motor unit recruitment) is not entirely fixed, though it tends to fall into certain patterns. In general, motor units in slow-twitch fibre (ST fibre, also known as 'red' or Type I fibre) are recruited more readily than those in fast-twitch (FT, 'white' or Type II) fibre, this having to do with the relative EMG potential amplitudes of the two types of fibre. Under certain conditions, however, it has been found that this firing order can be reversed, and that the more forceful, faster-contracting white units can be activated before, or even without, activation of the usually low-threshold units of red muscle.[14] These findings make it clear that the order of recruitment is determined, not within the motoneurons themselves, but in the synaptic inputs to them.[15]

The practical implications of these findings for weight training are worth consideration. Basmajian has found that motor learning and control are not a process of accretion (i.e. a process of adding more and more motor units) but rather the opposite—the inhibition of motor units that are not strictly required to perform the movement. 'Electromyographic studies in health and disease', he writes, 'indicate that the acquisition of skills occurs through the selective inhibition of unnecessary muscular activity rather than the activation of additional motor units'.[16] He quotes numerous experiments to show that, as a skill is learned, there is a marked reduction of activity in auxiliary muscles (known as synergists) while the activity of the main muscle, or prime mover, remains the same. Even more importantly from our present point of view, this process may occur within an individual muscle:

> Physiologists and even some kinesiologists do not appreciate that each and every muscle has several (sometimes many) component parts which are recruited in different functions at different times. Many investigations with intramuscular electrodes in many thousands of muscles lead me to believe that this local activity is patterned by progressive inhibition of motoneurons until an acceptable performance is achieved.[17]

In the light of this evidence, it can be seen that one of the effects of training is to localise more and more precisely the areas of muscle which are called into vigorous action by the performance of a task or movement.

This notion is borne out by research which has been devoted to the specificity of training effects associated with different kinds of training. It is well established, for instance, that isometric training can cause a significant increase in isometric contraction strength at the joint positions trained, but may cause no significant increase at 'unfamiliar' joint angles. Conversely, isotonic training (concentric and eccentric contractions) causes a large increase in weight-lifting strength but not in isometric strength. There is a similar opposition between isometric and isokinetic training,[18] such that increases in isokinetic strength are not replicated by increases in isometric strength and vice versa. Each particular form of training tends to be highly specific in its effect.

The implications of this 'specificity theory' for muscle fibre recruitment are highly significant, not only in terms of strength and motor learning but also in respect of muscular development. They can best be summarised in the words of Digby G. Sale:

> The recruitment order of motor units is rather fixed for a muscle involved in a specific movement, even if the rate of force development or speed of contraction varies (Desmedt & Godeaux, 1977). However, in the case of a change in position (Person, 1974) or in the case of a multifunction muscle performing different movements (Desmedt & Godeaux, 1981; Haar Romeny, Dernier Van Der Gon, & Gielen, 1982; Schmidt & Thomas, 1981), recruitment order can be altered. Thus, some motor units within a muscle might have a low threshold for one movement and a higher threshold for another movement. The variation in recruitment order according to movement may be partially responsible for the specificity of training that has been observed (Sale & MacDougall, 1981) and may support the notion long held by strength trainers that full development of a muscle is possible only when it is exercised in all its possible movements.[19]

The relevance of this observation is best seen against the background that weight training is most fully effective when it comes closest to activating the greatest possible number of muscle motor units. It is a well-attested finding that trainers with the greatest muscular development are the most capable of activating all muscle fibres by voluntary contraction.[20]

It has been suggested that the neural inhibition which makes it difficult to activate all motor units is a form of 'natural protection': if untrained muscles were capable of truly maximal contractions, they could be more subject to injury through infrequent strong exertion. Even in advanced trainers, the ability to achieve full muscle activation not infrequently results in a muscle being torn or even ripped from its attachments. In such cases, the untrained person's inability to activate all motor units acts as a kind of protection by making the maximum exertion impossible (i.e., the weight cannot be lifted in the first place).

The Matrix System addresses the question of full fibre activation without the use of the heavy weights that are likely to lead to injury. In *The Matrix Principle*, we referred to what we called 'deep fibre activation', the process whereby 'a comprehensive growth response can be achieved by combining a range of specific movements designed to tax the muscle from different angles and in varying modes within a systematic framework of progressive resistance'.[21] By exploiting more fully than other training systems the range of different movements, part-movements and isometric tensions of which the muscles are capable, Matrix training activates a greater number of motor units including those whose threshold of activity is not reached by the more limited recruitment effects of conventional training.

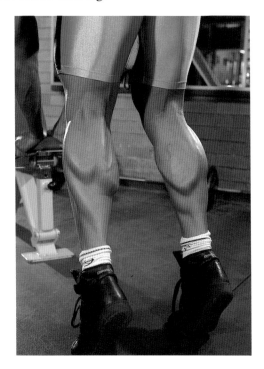

The phenomenal calf development of Jamie Roberts.

Muscle contraction

The response of muscle to various forms of exertion is an *adaptive* response; that is, the muscle alters its characteristics to enable it to respond more effectively to the type of exertion involved. Broadly, it may adapt by increasing either its endurance capacity or its force capacity, or in some cases both. In the case of endurance, adaptation usually involves improvement in the aerobic enzyme systems of ST (or Type I) muscle associated with increased oxidative capacity and more and larger capillaries. In the case of improved force, the adaptation is in terms of increased contractile strength and increase in muscle size. Training-induced hypertrophy (an increase in muscle cross-sectional area) tends to be greater in FT (or Type II) fibre than in ST fibre, though both types of fibre show some adaptive response as measured by growth in cross-sectional area. In a study by MacDougall where the triceps were trained for a period of 5–6 months, the area of Type II fibre was found to have increased by 33 per cent and that of Type I fibre by 27 per cent.[22]

There is an obvious association between an increase in strength and an increase in muscle bulk, as witness the fact that heavyweight weight-lifters can lift more than those in lighter divisions; nonetheless, the relationship between increase in strength and increase in bulk is not linear—a fact which gives rise to the popular misconception that the muscles of bodybuilders are not actually strong. They are, however, very strong indeed compared with those of the 'average' person, though not necessarily as strong as those of elite weight-lifters. The difference is largely a function of the specificity of training methods used, the weight-lifter's relying more on single repetitions at great weight rather than on multiple reps at sub-maximal loadings. Overall, there are strong correlations between force output and muscle cross-sectional area, such that the observations made above on strength development are also generally relevant to muscle growth or hypertrophy.

An increase in the size of muscles is not, however, the only anabolic or growth-related effect of strength training. Training-induced hypertrophy of muscle fibres is generally accompanied by a proportional increase in connective tissue, so that the thickness of ligaments and tendons grows at the same rate as the muscle itself. The proportion of non-contractile tissue to muscle tends to remain the same in all individuals regardless of muscle size or state of training, so that the absolute amount of connective tissue is considerably greater in bodybuilders than in untrained subjects.[23] This adaptation is clearly necessary in order to enable the muscles to exert more force without undue strain or damage to surrounding tissue. One of the problems with anabolic steroid use is that it increases muscle fibre growth at a rate greater than that at which the related connective tissue growth occurs. It seems likely that this is a significant factor in the increased incidence of muscle tears amongst steroid users.

In *The Matrix Principle*, we described the structure of muscle fibre, noting that it can be analysed or broken down into progressively smaller components: initially into what are called fibrils (or myofibrils, literally 'muscle fibrils'), then into still smaller units known as filaments (or myofilaments). Myofilaments are made up of two components, actin and myosin, and the shortening and 'bunching' of muscle fibres which occur with contraction result from the sliding together of actin and myosin components—a process usually described by what is known as the sliding filament theory (see *The Matrix Principle*, p.17). The process has been described in detail by Langley et al.:

> The mechanism responsible for the sliding of the filaments over one another is now fairly well understood. In brief, the heads of the myosin molecules attach to points on the actin molecules, then bend so as to pull the actin molecules with them. The heads now disengage from the actin molecules, bend back to their former position, reattach to actin, and bend once again. It is very similar to rowing a boat, except that the myosin molecules do not work in unison. Each stroke by a myosin pulls an actin molecule only a short distance, but by virtue of a series of rapid strokes by a great many myosins, muscle shortening occurs.[24]

When attached to the actin filament, the myosin head is referred to as a *cross-bridge*.

The effect of repeated contraction under tension is an increase in the contractile protein content of the muscle resulting from the addition of actin and myosin filaments. Just how this process occurs is not yet fully known, some physiologists claiming to have discovered an increase in the numbers of myosin filaments relative to actin. Clarke, for instance, refers to work done by Penman in 1970 on progressive resistance exercise in college athletes, as a result of which

> . . . muscle biopsies revealed increased myosin filament concentration, a reduction in the distance between myosin filaments, and fewer actin filaments in orbit around a myosin filament. In other words, there would seem to be an increase in the packing density of the interdigitating filaments within a cell, plus a changing ratio of actin to myosin.[25]

On the other hand, MacDougall's studies on the packing density of the myosin filaments revealed no such effect: 'The spacing of the myosin filaments was found to be extremely consistent within each subject and between each condition [trained and immobilised muscles]'.[26] MacDougall's view is that 'because the packing density of the myosin filaments remains the same at the interior of the myofibril as at the exterior, it is apparent that the contractile proteins are added to the outside of the myofibril and thus do not alter the cross-bridge configurations'.[27] The fact that myofibril cross-sectional area increased significantly (by 16 per cent) following training and decreased by a similar amount following immobilisation is attributed by MacDougall to the 'splitting' of myofibrils:

> Goldspink (1970) has suggested several mechanisms by which this splitting process might occur, including a mechanical possibility related to discrepancies between the A and I band lattice spacing. Because of this discrepancy, with contraction, the peripheral I filaments (actin) are pulled at an angle slightly oblique to the myofibril axis. As more filaments are added to the myofibril, the girth and strength are increased and the strain causes the center of the Z discs to rupture, resulting in two or more 'daughter' myofibrils of the same sarcomere length.[28]

The increases in muscle fibre size resulting from contraction are seen, in this view, as being due to changes in myofibril number as well as myofibril size—a view supported by the finding that, with training, total fibre area increased by a greater proportion than did myofibril area.

The above discussion may seem academic, but it serves to indicate the extent to which our knowledge of the muscle hypertrophy mechanism is limited and how far we still have to go in understanding the precise nature of the training stimulus. It is certainly clear that the effect of certain types of training is to foster the production of additional contractile protein (actin and myosin), and that this can only be done by a series of 'messages' conveyed through the body's cells. (Our 'blueprint' DNA sends a messenger RNA into the muscle fibre where constituent amino acids are gathered and positioned by transfer RNA to form the protein.) But the exact relationship between the mechanical process of contraction and the biological process of protein production remains the subject of ongoing research.

Broadly, two main hypotheses have emerged in research on muscle hypertrophy. The first, which might be termed the 'direct action' hypothesis, suggests that muscle tension is the key that provides the signal for increased uptake of amino acids and enhanced synthesis of contractile protein through increased RNA activity. This theory is supported by the evidence that a high degree of tension causes a hyperpolarisation of the muscle cell which facilitates amino acid transport, and causes the release of prostaglandin F2 which accelerates protein synthesis and decreases protein degradation.[29] The second proposed explanation, which we may call the 'indirect action' hypothesis, is closer to the conventional belief that intensive training breaks down protein which is then rebuilt in larger quantities (a process referred to as 'overcompensation') between training sessions.

In support of this second view, researchers point to signs of damage in contractile protein and connective tissue following training (e.g. leakage of the muscle enzyme creatine kinase, the presence of myoglobin in the urine, and elevations in urinary hydroxyproline) and suggest that the repeated process of damage and repair may result in an overshoot of protein synthesis similar to the overcompensation of muscle glycogen that occurs in response to endurance training.[30] Karpovich and Sinning, for example, point out that overcompensation is a common response to the loss of organic material from the body:

> Examples of the law of overcompensation are seen in the production of antitoxin and other immunizing substances, [when] the body is subjected to the action of disease-producing toxins, or in the development of callus on the palm of the hand as the result of friction and pressure which remove the superficial layers of the skin.[31]

They conclude that the growth of muscle must be 'in some way linked with the destruction of constituents of the muscle that takes place during strenuous muscular contraction'.[32]

Although scientific evidence has been advanced in support of both the above hypotheses, definitive conclusions have yet to be reached and must await further studies.

Training and muscle growth

In the absence of definitive scientific answers to the questions discussed above, our best practical approach to the issues they raise is to examine as closely as possible the empirical links between training *methods* and training *outcomes*. In this way, we may at least turn to good use the scientific evidence we already have, even if more detail is yet to be discovered as to the manner in which the outcomes are produced. Let us consider, for example, the typical effects of the three most common forms of weight training, known as *isotonic*, *isometric* and *isokinetic* training.

Briefly stated, isotonic training consists of the repeated lifting and lowering of a weight or other form of resistance. The term is applied to the use of both free weights and machines where the training effect derives from the concentric and eccentric movement of limbs by the progressive contraction and relaxation of the muscles.

Isometric training was popular in the 1950s and 1960s, but is less used nowadays, largely because the claims initially made for it proved to be exaggerated. The isometric method consists of holding a weight (or maintaining resistance) in a stationary position for a given period, so that the muscles are maximally contracted but the muscle-lever system performs no work. It has been shown in some tests to produce significant gains in strength (perhaps because of the triggering effect of oxygen deficit resulting from compression of the muscle capillaries), but these gains are specific to the joint-angle exercised. To effect strength gains throughout the full range of motion, many different joint-angles need to be trained.

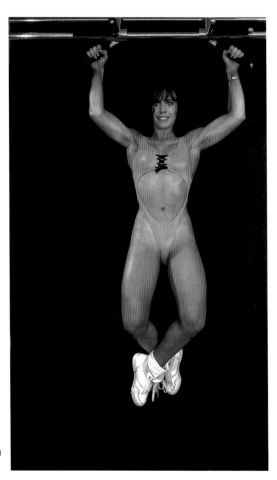

Tracey Moonen shows her form with
Matrix Chin-Ups.

Isokinetic training (or accommodating resistance exercise) was developed in order to overcome one of the main deficiencies in conventional isotonic training. In an isotonic contraction, the main muscle (or prime mover) involved is stronger at some points in the movement than at others, because the mechanical advantage at which it is working varies from one point to another of the lift. Thus, an isotonic lift can be done in strict fashion (i.e. without using momentum) only with a weight that the muscle can move at its weakest point in the lift; conversely, at stronger points, the weight that is being lifted is less than what is needed for near-maximal activation of the muscle.

Isokinetic training must be done on machines specifically designed for the purpose, which hold the speed of contraction constant and thus apply a high force at all times during the movement. Isokinetic work has been found in controlled tests to be a highly effective training method in those applications for which machines are available,[33] though the latter tend to be expensive and some do not provide eccentric loading which means that they lose the advantage provided by a combination of concentric and eccentric contractions.[34] A number of experienced weight instructors also consider that machines (especially when these are the sole or main training device used) unduly restrict the range of movement and thus fail to exploit fully the activity of the exercising limbs through all their parameters of motion.

Each of the three exercise methods described has specific merits, and some disadvantages, compared with the others. Attempts have been made to combine the characteristics of more than one of them, as in the method known as functional isometrics in which a weight is lifted and held against an immovable object for several counts. This combination of isometric and dynamic training has been found by sports physiologists to produce the advantages of both forms.[35]

Matrix training goes further than any other method in combining the positive features of isotonic, isometric and isokinetic exercise. Like functional isometrics, it incorporates elements of isometric and dynamic training, but by constantly changing the joint-angles of isometric holding it overcomes the point-specific limitations inherent in conventional isometric training which tends to be restricted to the midpoint of muscular contractions. Additionally, although the biomechanics of Matrix training differ from those of isokinetic exercise, it achieves a similar effect by ensuring that the muscles are fully worked at all levels of mechanical advantage and disadvantage. By stopping the movement at various points of the range of motion, Matrix training prevents the use of momentum to carry the weight through its sticking point (the area of maximum mechanical disadvantage). By stressing the muscle at the points of axis at which its leverage advantage is minimised, it isolates the points of greatest vulnerability and weakness within the arc of movement and thus places more significant demands on the muscle than can be achieved (even with heavier weight) by conventional isotonic exercise. Moreover, by using both eccentric and concentric contractions, Matrix training overcomes the limitations of those forms of isokinetic apparatus which use concentric contractions alone.

Although the end points of a Matrix movement are the same as those of conventional isotonic exercise—the point of maximal stretch or extension (the starting point) and that of maximal contraction (the finishing point)—it will be seen that the point at which the Matrix movement characteristically differs from the conventional isotonic movement is that point along the arc of movement where the weight is held either momentarily or for an isometric contraction. The change from a concentric to an eccentric contraction (sometimes separated by isometric holding) occurs, depending on the exercise, at one or more positions along the arc of movement, which means that most of the ergonomic work is done at these positions rather than at the end points of the movement.

The advantage of the Matrix contraction pattern can be understood in terms of the sliding filament theory of muscle contraction. As Langley et al. put it:

> If the muscle is stretched to the point where there is little or no overlap of the myosin and actin filaments, the ability of the muscle to contract will be minimal. At the other extreme, that is, when the muscle is approaching maximal contraction, the ends of the actin filaments are seen to overlap. This is, again, a very inefficient arrangement which would diminish the force of contraction. Between these two extremes the cross-bridges are organized in such a way that provides the power for the greatest force of contraction of which the muscle is capable'.[36]

Matrix exercise thus concentrates the muscular effort more exclusively in the area of contraction at which actin-myosin interaction is at its maximum, producing an intensity of training effect far greater than is achieved by the use of conventional isotonic repetitions.

The capacity of Matrix training to maximise the *intensity* of resistance-based exercise, even with the use of light weights, is a crucial element of its enhanced effectiveness in stimulating the process of muscle growth, and the above discussion may suggest some of the physiological basis for the superior results it has demonstrated in controlled comparisons with conventional methods. In the next chapter, we shall set out the main principles which trainers should apply in their workout regime in order to optimise their capacity for muscle growth through the use of Matrix training regimes.

References

1   J.D. MacDougall, 'Morphological changes in human skeletal muscle following strength training and immobilization', in *Human Muscle Power* (Proceedings of a Symposium on Human Muscle Power at McMaster University, Canada, in 1984), N.L. Jones et al. eds, Human Kinetics Publishers, Inc., Champaign, Ill, 1986, p. 281.
2   See Brian J. Sharkey, *Physiology of Fitness*, Human Kinetics Books, Champaign, Ill, 3rd ed. 1990, p. 74.

3   Tests reported by Digby G. Sale, 'Neural adaptations in strength and power training', in *Human Muscle Power*, p. 290.
4   See Peter G. Bursztyn, *Physiology for Sportspeople: A Serious User's Guide to the Body*, Manchester University Press, Manchester & New York, 1990, p. 27.
5   See Sale, 'Neural adaptations ...' p. 295.
6   See J.V.Basmajian, *Muscles Alive: Their Functions Revealed by Electromyography*, Williams & Wilkins, Baltimore, 4th ed. 1979, p. 108.
7   See Sale, 'Neural adaptations ...' p. 291.
8   ibid., p. 289.
9   See Michael H. Stone & Harold S. O'Bryant, *Weight Training: A Scientific Approach*, Burgess International (Bellwether Press), Edina, MN, 1987, p. 10.
10 Sale, 'Neural adaptations...' p. 291.
11 Basmajian, *Muscles Alive*, p. 126.
12 Basmajian, *Muscles Alive*, p. 126.
13 ibid., p. 7, p. 9.
14 See Basmajian, *Muscles Alive*, p. 16; cf. MacDougall, 'Morphological changes...' pp. 15–16.
15 See MacDougall, 'Morphological, changes...' Basmajian, *Muscles Alive*, pp. 15-16.
16 Basmajian, *Muscles Alive*, p. 106.
17 ibid., p. 107.
18 See Sharkey, *Physiology of Fitness*, p. 76.
19 Sale, 'Neural adaptations...' p. 298.
20 See Peter V. Karpovich & Wayne E. Sinning, *Physiology of Muscular Activity*, W.B. Saunders, Philadelphia/London/Toronto 7th ed. 1971, p. 28.
21 Ronald S. Laura & Kenneth R. Dutton, *The Matrix Principle*, Allen & Unwin, Sydney, 1991, p. 126.
22 See MacDougall, 'Morphological changes...' p. 271.
23 ibid., p. 279.
24 L.L. Langley, Ira R. Telford & John B. Christensen, *Dynamic Anatomy and Physiology*, McGraw-Hill, New York, 5th ed. 1980, p. 128.
25 David H. Clarke, *Exercise Physiology*, Prentice-Hall Inc., Englewood Cliffs, N.J.1975, p. 51.
26 MacDougall, 'Morphological changes...' p. 273.
27 MacDougall, 'Morphological changes...'p. 273.
28 MacDougall, 'Morphological changes...', pp. 274–5.
29 ibid., p. 281.
30 See MacDougall, 'Morphological changes...', p. 281 cf. Sharkey, *Physiology of Fitness*, p.80.
31 Karpovich & Sinning, *Physiology of Muscular Activity*, p. 21.
32 ibid., p. 20.
33 See Clarke, *Exercise Physiology*, p. 49.
34 See Stone & O'Bryant, *Weight Training*, p. 110.
35 See ibid., p. 147.
36 See Langley et al., *Dynamic Anatomy*, pp. 134-5.

2   How to use Matrix training

To gain the optimum benefit from Matrix training, the routines need to be performed in the manner for which they were designed; that is, as a form of *high-intensity* training. As Matrix differs in this respect from most other forms of weight training, it is important at the outset to understand the concept of high intensity on which it is based before going on to look at how this training method can be incorporated into the workout regime.

According to the principle known as SAID (Specific Adaptation to Imposed Demands), the body reacts in quite specific ways to the demands that are made upon it by *adapting* in order to cope with these demands more easily. The body's adaptive capacity is obviously limited in absolute terms: it will, for example, differ from one individual to another according to the constraints imposed by our genetics—the innate capacity of our DNA to send the necessary messages to the body's constituent cells. It may also vary from time to time within a single individual depending on factors such as age and the general fitness or state of health of the body. Diet, sex, previous training experience and a number of other variables also affect our adaptive capacity.

Notwithstanding these variations, each of us reacts to a repeated physical demand for which our body's protective margins are inadequate. We do this either by succumbing under the demand—if it is beyond our responsive capacity—or by altering our body's physical and metabolic status so as to meet the demand and thus restore equilibrium to the system. The reaction, clearly, needs to be both specific to, and proportionate to, the imposed demand in order to be effective.

In the case of weight or resistance training, we noted in chapter 1 that the body's reactions to various training modes tend to be highly specific, and that clear differentials in, for example, strength gains have been observed by exercise physiologists between subjects who have undergone periods of isotonic, isometric or isokinetic training. Considerable care is needed in measuring such differences, to ensure that the training stimulus is comparable, in the case of each method tested, in terms of such variables as duration of training sessions, their frequency, the body parts or strength

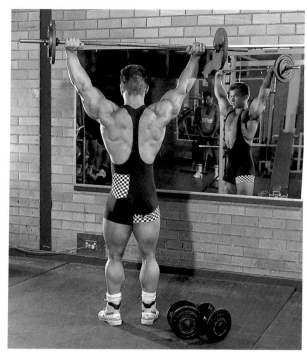

The extraordinary back of
Lee Priest.

functions targeted, non-exercise factors involved, and the like. With these
provisos, it is possible to determine with reasonable accuracy the typical
effect of training modes on the adaptive mechanisms of skeletal muscle.

Along with these differences in specificity of response, weight training
also elicits various responses in individuals depending upon the intensity of
the stimulus. Conventional isotonic exercise, for example, tends to be
relatively ineffective unless the weight used is between 75 per cent and 80
per cent of the maximum which an individual can lift for a single repetition
(RM); below this level, training may have some aerobic effect but has little
impact upon muscular growth. For this reason, the low weight, repetitive
isotonic movements used in 'circuit training' may be of assistance in some
forms of athletic training, but are not of any real value for those wishing
to add to their muscle bulk. Conversely, low repetitions at maximum weight
(as in powerlifting) have been found to increase strength and power, but
they appear to affect fast-twitch fibre predominantly[1] whereas more repetitions at lower weight affect not only fast but also the slow fibre whose
selective hypertrophy has been found to be characteristic of world-class
bodybuilders.[2] As distinct from the other effects of weight training (strength
and endurance gain), its specifically hypertrophic effect is thus dependent
on that combination of resistance-force and pattern of repetitive contraction
which will elicit the optimum degree of sustained intensity, and is the point
at which the volume or intensity of stimulus is kept as high as possible
without its resulting in the overwork which may cause injury and would
adversely affect recovery ability.[3]

High-intensity exercise is aimed at achieving this optimal effect by max-imising the intensity of response of the muscles to the contraction stimulus rather than by simply increasing the amount of the stimulus. For continued muscle adaptation, an overload must constantly exist; that is, a load which cannot be lifted without a high degree of stress on the muscle. As the muscles grow stronger, the same workload is not registered as being of high intensity and the stimulus must be increased. The response of conventional isotonic exercise is to increase the load, but this is effective only up to the point at which the load can no longer be lifted because the trainer's maximum strength level has been reached. High-intensity exercise, on the other hand, achieves the overload effect by making the muscles work as hard as possible for a given weight, limiting their capacity to accommodate the weight through neural adaptation, movement anticipation, momentum and recovery pauses. By this means, the muscles are forced to call upon all their reserves in order to maintain the required response: more and more muscle fibres must be brought into play as the assistance of other support systems (neurological, biomechanical and physiological) is minimised. As the trainer becomes more and more able to cope with these demands, the intensity with which they are imposed is further increased by more and more difficult contraction patterns, reduced pauses, and (within the much stricter parameters of an intense routine) some increase in weight.

In the following sections, we shall examine the practical implications of the high-intensity training method and suggest how they should be incor-porated in the workout regime.

Cadence

The cadence (i.e. number of isotonic reps per minute) used in Matrix training is similar to that usually recommended for isotonic training generally—though of course this applies only to the concentric and eccentric move-ments, not to the isometric holding included in some routines (for which the number of seconds of 'holding' is specified in the routine itself). A rate of approximately 60 reps per minute—one rep per second—should be the aim: this rate can best be achieved by counting to yourself 'A thousand and one, a thousand and two' etc., at each rep.

If repetitions are performed too quickly, momentum will inevitably be used (particularly on the full repetitions) and the muscles will not be fully brought into play. On the other hand, Matrix is not designed to be performed as a form of super-slow training, as fatigue will set in too quickly and the trainer's ability to perform the full routines set out will be impaired.

The high-intensity training effect derives primarily from maintaining a continuous motion in the isotonic repetitions, and not pausing between reps. Research studies have shown that raising the intercontraction rest period so that relaxation occurs between contractions allows recuperation to occur and thus diminishes the high intensity of the stimulus. In a series of experiments by D.H. Clarke[4] the level of 'steady state' strength at 60 reps per minute for six minutes was 20 kg; dropping the reps to 45 per minute raised the steady state to 25 kg, while 30 reps per minute raised it further to 31 kg and 15 reps per minute to 45 kg. To put this another way, it could be concluded that a weight lifted at 15 reps per minute (i.e. with approximately 3 seconds recuperation between repetitions) would have to be more than twice the weight lifted at a one-second cadence (60 reps per minute, without pauses) in order to have the same effect on the muscles. For this reason, high-intensity work with no pauses between reps is able to make use of relatively lighter weights.

Pauses between sets

The high-intensity effect also relies on minimising the pauses between sets. To eliminate the pauses completely would be counter productive, as once fatigue has set in it cannot be overcome until the 'strength debt' has been repaid to a sufficient degree to allow the muscles to continue work at adequate capacity. Continuing to work muscles which have become fatigued results in a reduced capacity to recruit muscle fibre; as Stone and O'Bryant put it:

> This method of training [one set to exhaustion] greatly reduces the workload made possible by multiple sets, which means the activated motor units receive less training. Part of the reason behind using sets to exhaustion is that, due to fatigue, the nth repetition would be maximal using an RM repetition scheme. This confuses relative and absolute maximum tensions; fatigue inhibits the use of some fibers, whereas all fibers are active with absolute maximum tension. Tension, not fatigue, is the major factor in developing maximum strength.[5]

On the other hand, if each set fully activated the muscle fibres, there would be no need for multiple sets; one set (whether to exhaustion or not) would suffice for each movement. Clearly this is not the case, and the reasoning behind multiple sets is that each set should build upon the set preceding it.

What is necessary, then, is a pause between sets which is sufficient to allow not complete recovery but *some* recovery to take place so that exhaustion is avoided. Complete recovery would mean that the next set had no more effect than that preceding it, whereas substantial but incomplete recovery means that the following set, even with the same weight, requires a slightly greater response from the muscle fibres than the set preceding. In this way, more and more motor units are recruited and maximum tension is maintained rather than the fall-off in fibre recruitment that results from fatigue.

The recovery process is in fact remarkably rapid: in isotonic exercise, 72 per cent recovery takes place within the first minute and more than 50 per cent within the first 30 seconds.[6] As a form of high-intensity exercise, Matrix training takes advantage of this rapid recovery process, specifying various lengths of pause between sets and groups of sets. The length of pause depends upon the difficulty of the exercise and the level at which it is performed, so that in some cases there is as little as a 30-second pause (meaning that the next set will be performed at something over 50 per cent of the recovery level). By two to three minutes a steady state has again been activated, resulting in no further gains from this component of the recovery process, and for this reason there are longer pauses specified between groups of sets so that the next group begins at full strength.

(There is another, slower, component of the recovery process, which is not complete until several hours after the cessation of exercise,[7] but this is of most importance in the heightened metabolic rate which follows vigorous exercise than in the motor unit recruitment effect of the exercise bout itself. This issue is discussed in detail in *The Matrix Principle*, pp. 49–50.)

It is therefore important, in performing Matrix exercise, to note carefully the length of pauses between sets and groups of sets, and to perform the routines according to this schedule. Any increase in the pauses will inevitably detract to some extent from the high-intensity effect and thus reduce the effectiveness of the Matrix routine.

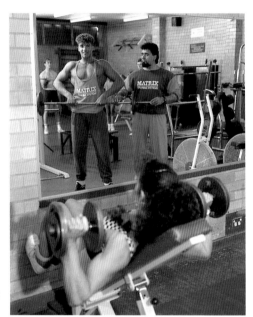

Professor Laura demonstrates the Matrix principle to one of his trainees.

Weight

No particular weight is, or can be, specified for the various routines given below. Much obviously depends on each individual's strength level, age, sex and training experience, and those who have not previously undertaken Matrix training will need to experiment for a short period before determining what is their beginning weight for each particular exercise.

As a rule of thumb, we suggest that those who are new to Matrix training begin each exercise using approximately 40 per cent of the weight that they can lift for a single repetition of the movement specified. Thus, if you can bench press 90 kg (200 lb) for a single rep, you would attempt the first Matrix bench press exercise with 40 per cent of that weight (90 kg x .40 = 36 kg or 80 lb). If you can perform the routine easily with this weight—you feel little or no degree of challenge to the muscles or can sense that they have not reached their maximum degree of tension by the end of the exercise (assuming it is performed strictly and as specified)—then your beginning weight was too low. You should pause for two to three minutes, load another 5 kg (or 10 lb) on the bar, and perform the exercise again, repeating this process if necessary until you reach sufficient weight to challenge the relevant muscles to the maximum. Conversely, if your beginning weight was such that you could not complete the first exercise as specified, or had to pause in the middle of a continuous set, you should wait for a few minutes and try again with less weight on the bar.

Your first Matrix workout (or the first for each body part) may thus be a process of trial and error, until you have found your appropriate beginning weight for each exercise. As individual beginning weights may differ even between similar exercises—for example barbell curls and incline dumbbell curls—it will be important for you to make a note of these in your training diary so that you do not need to rely on memory when you next work the same body part.

Once you have determined your beginning weights, you will need to concentrate on performing the exercises in strict *form*; that is, with the minimum assistance from synergist or 'aiding' muscles, and on careful observance of the short pauses specified. This point cannot be stressed too strongly. You may well be able to complete the programme of routines in the number of weeks prescribed and may congratulate yourself on doing so, but if you have done so only by sacrificing form or by compromising the recommended pause periods between the sets, then the regrettable truth is that you have not really been performing high-intensity Matrix exercise at all, and have been cheating only one person—yourself.

Assuming, however, that you are working to strict form and to the pauses specified, you will find that as your body accustoms itself to the Matrix regime your beginning weight is no longer sufficient to maintain the maximum challenge to the muscle system, and that you need to make progressive, though gradual, additions to the weights with which you began. Progression is an important component of any weight programme, and is the chief factor involved in maintaining the overload required to promote the adaptive response on the part of the muscle system.

As mentioned above, Matrix training relies less than other systems on a constant increase in weight. As you progress through the Matrix routines set out below, the increasing difficulty of the exercise pattern which occurs from one twelve-week schedule to the next will play the major part in keeping up the necessary overload on the muscle system; nonetheless, depending to some extent on individual capacity and speed of muscular adaptation, trainers will also find that increases in weight are also needed from time to time in order to maintain the intensity of the training effect.

No trainer who has been working conscientiously will be content to remain at the beginning weight, and the majority will wish to add to their weight periodically as training continues.

It should be noted that, because of its high intensity, Matrix training requires that only *small* increments of weight be added in order to effect a marked increase in overload. For this reason, most trainers will find that the addition of 2.5 kg (5 lb) to the weight will be sufficient to transform a routine that has become relatively easy to perform into an intense stimulus which places exacting demands on the muscles involved. While such small increments might have little effect in conventional training, their impact is magnified by the contraction patterns that characterise Matrix exercise, and large increases in weight are not only unnecessary but will be found impossible to manage.

Overall, however, priority should be given to performing the Matrix routines strictly and in accordance with instructions, moving through the programme from less difficult to more demanding routines. Only when this is being done and the weight is still found to be insufficient should it be increased. This difference between Matrix and conventional training is fundamental to gaining the maximum benefit from the Matrix System.

Frequency of workouts

The four twelve-week training schedules set out in chapter 3 of this book are intended primarily as a *guide* for trainers: they are not meant to lock them into a training regimen which is fixed once and for all and cannot be varied. Some degree of experimentation is not only desirable but is, in fact, essential if you are to tailor your Matrix training to the individual needs and capability of your own muscle system.

With this important proviso, we have set out below a schedule which should suit most trainers. You will note that it provides a four-day weekly training programme in which each major body part is worked twice per week. The training days and free days are varied from week to week, but some adjustment can be made to this schedule depending on your preferences and your other commitments. The years of clinical trials which have gone into the development of the Matrix System have shown this type of exercise pattern to produce the best gains.

Some very advanced trainers may, at least in some weeks, train the same body part up to three times in the course of a week. Such cases are quite exceptional, however, and would comprise mainly competitive bodybuilders and a small number of others whose bodies are able to cope with the high intensity of Matrix exercise to an unusually high degree. For most trainers, even those who have considerable muscle mass, it will be advisable to train each major body part only twice per week.

Again, we stress that this advice is meant as a guide only. Once you have followed the recommended training schedule for at least a six-week period, you should know whether you are taking too much or too little recuperation time. If your nutritional intake is sufficient but you are feeling continually fatigued, find that your muscles are not holding their pump as usual, and come from one workout to the next with sore muscles, there is a good chance that you are overtraining. If this happens, you can either diminish the intensity of your Matrix workout or increase the number of recuperation days per week.On the other hand, if at the end of six weeks you find that you are not working hard enough and have more than sufficient energy to spare, you may wish to use a scheduled free day to train a particular body part which would otherwise have been trained on another day in that week, or to concentrate on a particular muscle group which needs more attention.

You will note that in the twelve-week schedule set out over the following pages the abdominal and calf specialisation routines have been incorporated into the core programme. The forearm specialisation routines can be added to any of the daily exercise routines or, alternatively, they can be introduced on the free days. You can thus adapt the programme to meet your individual needs and training level.

WEEK 1

Monday	Tuesday	Wednesday	Thursday	Friday	Saturday	Sunday
Chest + Deltoids + Abdominals	Biceps + Triceps	Free day	Legs + Lats & back + Calves	Free day	Triceps + Chest + Abdominals	Free day

WEEK 2

Monday	Tuesday	Wednesday	Thursday	Friday	Saturday	Sunday
Biceps + Lats & back + Abdominals	Legs + Triceps + Calves	Free day	Chest + Deltoids + Abdominals	Free day	Legs + Lats & back + Abdominals	Free day

WEEK 3

Monday	Tuesday	Wednesday	Thursday	Friday	Saturday	Sunday
Triceps + Chest + Abdominals	Free day	Legs + Deltoids + Calves	Biceps + Triceps + Abdominals	Free day	Chest + Lats & back + Abdominals	Free day

WEEK 4

Monday	Tuesday	Wednesday	Thursday	Friday	Saturday	Sunday
Legs + Lats & back + Calves	Free day	Chest + Deltoids + Abdominals	Free day	Biceps + Triceps + Abdominals	Free day	Legs + Chest + Calves

WEEK 5

Monday	Tuesday	Wednesday	Thursday	Friday	Saturday	Sunday
Free day	Biceps + Triceps + Abdominals	Free day	Chest + Lats & back + Abdominals	Free day	Legs + Deltoids + Calves	Free day

WEEK 6

Monday	Tuesday	Wednesday	Thursday	Friday	Saturday	Sunday
Chest + Deltoids + Abdominals	Free day	Legs + Lats & back + Calves	Free day	Biceps + Triceps + Abdominals	Deltoids + Chest + Abdominals	Free day

WEEK 7

Monday	Tuesday	Wednesday	Thursday	Friday	Saturday	Sunday
Biceps + Lats & back + Abdominals	Legs + Triceps + Calves	Free day	Chest + Deltoids + Abdominals	Free day	Legs + Lats & back + Calves	Free day

WEEK 8

Monday	Tuesday	Wednesday	Thursday	Friday	Saturday	Sunday
Chest + Deltoids + Abdominals	Free day	Biceps + Lats & back + Abdominals	Free day	Legs + Triceps + Calves	Free day	Chest + Lats & back + Abdominals

WEEK 9

Monday	Tuesday	Wednesday	Thursday	Friday	Saturday	Sunday
Free day	Legs + Deltoids + Calves	Free day	Chest + Triceps + Abdominals	Legs + Deltoids + Calves	Biceps + Lats & back + Abdominals	Free day

WEEK 10

Monday	Tuesday	Wednesday	Thursday	Friday	Saturday	Sunday
Legs + Lats & back + Calves	Free day	Chest + Deltoids + Abdominals	Free day	Biceps + Triceps + Abdominals	Free day	Chest + Lats & back + Abdominals

WEEK 11

Monday	Tuesday	Wednesday	Thursday	Friday	Saturday	Sunday
Legs + Lats & back + Calves	Biceps + Triceps + Abdominals	Free day	Chest + Deltoids + Abdominals	Free day	Legs + Triceps + Calves	Free day

WEEK 12

Monday	Tuesday	Wednesday	Thursday	Friday	Saturday	Sunday
Chest + Deltoids + Abdominals	Free day	Biceps + Triceps + Abdominals	Chest + Legs + Calves	Free day	Biceps + Triceps	Chest + Lats & back + Abdominals

References

1   See Sharkey, *Physiology of Fitness*, p. 75.
2   See Stone & O'Bryant, *Weight Training*, pp. 14–15.
3   ibid., p. 106.
4   See references in Clarke, *Exercise Physiology*, pp. 42–4.
5   Stone & O'Bryant, *Weight Training*, p. 109.
6   See Clarke, *Exercise Physiology*, p. 45.
7   Clarke, *Exercise Physiology*, p. 45

3 Diet and supplementation

The promotion of muscle hypertrophy is not a matter of exercise alone. Appropriate nutrition is a crucial element of the total training regime, just as it is vital for achieving and maintaining general health, energy and fitness. It is an unfortunate fact that many weight trainers either fail to analyse and, if necessary, modify their eating habits when they embark on their training programme, or else assume simplistically that by eating more of everything they will foster the growth of muscle mass. Neither of these strategies is effective, and they may even be counter productive. Trainers who pay no attention, or insufficient attention, to dietary intake are often led to conclude that their workout regime is ineffective because they are not gaining significant muscle mass; the problem lies not with the training itself but with their failure to provide the muscle system with the nutritional material on which it needs to call in response to the demands of training.

Along with the development of Matrix exercise techniques, various controlled trials have been conducted under the supervision of Professor R.S. Laura in which training method and frequency have been kept identical between matched training groups, with dietary intake, including the intake of supplements, being the sole variable. Nutritional diaries were maintained alongside training diaries by the subjects participating in these trials, and the progress of subjects in the different groups was compared over set periods, usually of twelve weeks but in some cases ranging over periods up to one year. The information provided in this section is based on the outcome of these trials.

In the first instance, it should be noted that while characteristic patterns of muscle growth do emerge from changes in eating habits, considerable variation is observable from one individual to another even when dietary intake and exercise method are practically identical. The reason for this variability is the difference in individual metabolic rates between one individual and another. Given identical food intake, some people gain weight quickly and others slowly. Thus, what may be an optimal training diet for one person may be inadequate for another.

The practical implication of this fact is that, in respect of diet, each trainer will need to experiment to at least some degree with different foods, meal habits and dietary supplements in order to determine which particular combination is optimal in terms of the metabolism of each individual. Those who have a high metabolic rate (i.e. who rapidly convert their food intake into energy) find that they require very large quantities of food simply to maintain any muscle mass they may have gained, since a high proportion of their food intake passes through their bodies unmetabolised. 'Fast metabolisers' thus tend to be 'slow gainers', and the converse equally applies. Given that exercise also stimulates metabolism, the more exercise we undertake the more energy we need in order to maintain our body state. This is good news for those slow metabolisers whose weight is excessive because their dietary intake exceeds what is required to maintain equilibrium and tends to be stored as fat, since they can use exercise to elevate their metabolism and in conjunction with reduced food intake bring their weight down. To influence the metabolism in the other direction, however—to modify the body's metabolic response so that it tends to build up protein (the anabolic process) rather than break it down (the catabolic process)—is much more difficult. One approach to this problem, through a monthly dietary regime known as 'protein loading', has been described in our book *The Matrix Principle* (pp. 68–73), and the positive feedback from a large number of slow gainers who have found protein loading effective encourages us to recommend it to those who experience this problem.

The reader is also referred to *The Matrix Principle* (pp. 55–68) for suggestions as to a healthy weight-reduction diet, and for a concise guide (pp. 73–77) to the protein sources available in a wide variety of common foods along with the percentages of protein absorbed and converted into muscle tissue from these sources. By way of general summary, the following may be found to be useful information for those trainers who—depending on their individual metabolism—need to make a special effort to gain weight (or 'bulk up'), lose weight (or 'get ripped') or maintain the weight they have gained.

Gaining weight

As mentioned above, exercise tends to elevate metabolism. It is quite common for serious athletes and bodybuilders to experience a gradual drop in weight resulting from increased energy expenditure. Others may find that while their weight is not actually dropping they are underweight and need to add bulk (in the form of muscle mass) to their physique. In simple terms, the strategy should be to ensure that you eat more (in terms of calories or kilojoules) than you expel, but to do so by consuming appropriate foods; that is, the energy sources most readily convertible into muscle protein. A filling, varied and (as far as possible) natural daily diet should be supplemented by foods high in caloric value such as:

- Nuts, seeds, grains, beans, fruits (fresh or dried) especially bananas, and fruit juices;
- Cheese, yoghurt, ice cream and milk (plenty of milk should be drunk);
- Red and white meats including fish.

Do not turn to concentrated sweets for extra carbohydrates, and do not stuff yourself at every meal. Rather than three very large meals each day, it is better to have six meals each day (three moderate meals and three snacks), allowing two to three hours between meals. Weight-gain supplements (see below) may be taken at the end of meals or between meals. Throughout the day, constantly nibble on fruit, raw carrots and sometimes nuts, and vary the volume of these snacks to meet your energy needs and stop hunger pangs.

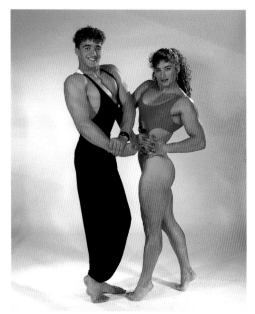

Teenage bench-press champion Adam
Laura with junior world champion,
Lin Mackie.

Losing weight

A combination of increased exercise and training is the best way to lose weight. Start a routine of aerobic exercise (swimming, running, cycling, home-exerciser biking). You may also find it helpful to replace one or two meals daily with a weight-loss preparation from a reputable manufacturer of diet supplements: this will allow you to lose weight without feeling 'empty' and debilitated.

Bodybuilders usually need to burn off some fat to improve their muscle definition for contests. The best way to do this is a little at a time, planning on losing no more than half to one kilogram (1–2 lb) of fat per week. If fat loss is achieved faster than this, it will usually be accompanied by a loss in muscle mass and in energy for training.

While you are dieting, you should increase your exercise. Some bodybuilders do this by a double-split routine, training twice a day, six days per week. Others practise quality training and add more aerobic exercises. When you walk or run a mile, you burn up about 419 kilojoules (about 100 calories); covering three miles three times per week will consume 3768 kilojoules (about 900 calories), in addition to the energy burned up in the gym. Even this level of energy expenditure is significant, particularly when added to your increased basal metabolic rate (which means that you burn more calories even during rest).

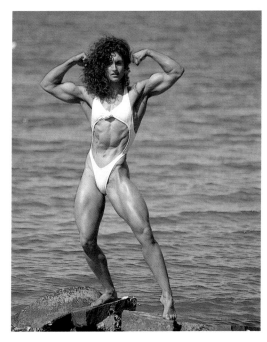

Lin Mackie shows her Matrix-built physique to great advantage.

Keeping steady weight

If you wish to maintain your weight, the following rough caloric estimates may be helpful:

- If you are inactive, multiply your weight (in pounds) by 10. This represents the number of calories you can take in over a 24-hour period to stay at even weight. If you weigh 91 kilograms (200 pounds), you can consume 8,374 kilojoules (2,000 calories) to maintain that weight;
- If you are moderately active—if, for instance, you play nine holes of golf three times a week, or play a couple of rounds of active tennis every week—you can safely consume about 15 times your weight in calories and stay at even weight. Thus, a person weighing 91 kilograms (200 pounds) can take in 12 560 kilojoules (3000 calories) over 24 hours;
- If you engage in strenuous physical activity every day, you can consume

up to 20 times your weight in calories and will probably still stay at even weight. Thus, a 91 kilogram (200 pound) bodybuilder who trains very hard (say, twice a day five times per week) can consume 16 747 kilojoules (4000 calories) a day and stay at even weight.

A simple kilojoule handbook available at the supermarket or newsagent, or the table in *The Matrix Principle* (pp. 73-7), will indicate the number of kilojoules (or calories) and the amount of protein, fats and carbohydrates, contained in various foods. Using this as a guide, and with appropriate balance between the four main food groups, you will be able to set up a suitable maintenance diet. Remember that the four main food groups are: the milk group (milk, cheese, cottage cheese); the meat group (also including fish, fowl, nuts, peas and beans); vegetables and fruits (including potatoes); breads and cereals (including rice and pasta).

Use of supplements

A balanced diet which draws upon a variety of food groups and has a bias towards natural (unprocessed) foods as far as possible or practical, is all that is required to provide the body with the essential elements required for growth. Many weight trainers will find that a daily food intake made up in this way will adequately cater for their nutritional needs. We acknowledge, however, that those trainers who seek to maximise their capacity for muscle gain usually find it helpful to supplement their regular meals by the use of various commercial products specifically formulated to complement and enhance the anabolic (or growth-producing) effects of the standard nutritional intake.

As with any other modification of the trainer's diet, the use of commercial supplements will vary in effectiveness from one trainer to another depending on individual metabolic capacity and other variables, which include such factors as genetic predisposition and basic body type (or somatotype). Most dietary supplements of the kind generally available in health stores or through bodybuilding and fitness magazines will not be found physically or psychologically harmful, and, if taken in accordance with directions, may often be useful in promoting muscle growth. Drugs such as anabolic steriods are not recommended for the initiation of muscle growth under any circumstances.

It should be noted, however, that the safety of some supposed 'muscle-building' products has been called into question. In particular, those containing L-tryptophan (which has been linked to the blood disease eosinophilia-myalgia syndrome) have now been banned from sale in the USA, and those containing gamma-hydroxybuteric acid are currently causing serious concern in medical circles. It is important to check the contents label to ensure that neither of these substances is included in any supplements you may take, just as it is important to check with your doctor (particularly if you are pregnant or suffer from high blood pressure) as to whether there are any substances—even those normally considered 'safe'—which you must carefully avoid. Moreover, some people are more sensitive than others to some of the components of diet supplements, and if you have the slightest suspicion of adverse side-effects caused by supplement use (even in small doses) you should discontinue their use immediately and seek medical advice.

These are important provisos, and what follows should be read with these warnings in mind. For most trainers, in our experience, the use of standard 'brand-name' supplements in recommended doses will not be found injurious to health; at worst, they may be found to have no significant anabolic effect. In this case, the only harm done will be to the wallet. The best advice which can be given to those thinking of embarking on a course of supplements is to do as much as possible to ensure that they take them under controlled conditions by maintaining their exercise regime and diet at normal levels, and comparing results over, say, a two-month period with and without supplements. (This will also allow you to monitor the supplement intake in terms of any adverse side-effects.) If there is no discernible difference in muscle growth, it may well be that your body's metabolism is not of a kind which responds positively to this form of supplementation, in which case you may wish to switch to a different type of supplement or discontinue supplement use entirely.

At the other end of the spectrum, however, lie those cases in which trainers have found commercial diet supplements to be of significant benefit in assisting or hastening increases in muscle mass. As part of the diet-testing programme accompanying the Matrix trials, a leading commercial brand of supplement was tested in a number of groups matched with control groups (all other variables being identical for all groups), and overall results suggested that the form of diet supplementation used was beneficial in fostering muscle growth.[1] This was the case in both Matrix and non-Matrix training groups, those trainers who used Matrix techniques with diet supplementation making, in most cases, even greater gains on the standard measures (see 'Introduction') than those using Matrix alone.

For those trainers wishing to use diet supplements, the best advice as to the amount required will be to follow the instructions given by the manufacturer. It is important not to exceed these dosages: not only does 'more' not mean 'better', but high toxicity levels can result from over-ingestion of certain substance components. Regrettably, warnings to this effect are not always given on container labels. Having made this point, it may be helpful here to give some indication as to how a conventional daily diet may be supplemented by commercially available products.

The two sample diets set out below are not meant to be followed slavishly, but are purely to suggest two quite different ways—among many possibilities—in which several 'meals' can be superimposed on the previous dietary regimen so as to match the trainer's workout programme. Here, two types of workout are given, the second being a split routine, to show the flexibility with which a daily schedule of meals and supplements can be organised.

DIET TYPE A

Breakfast (8.00 a.m.)
Four-egg cheese omelette
Whole-grain toast with butter
Piece of fresh fruit
Glass of non-fat milk
(Supplement—tablets)

Mid-morning (10.30 a.m.)
(Supplement—drink)

Lunch (1.00 p.m.)
Tuna salad (or roast beef) sandwich
Piece of fresh fruit
Glass of milk
(Supplement—tablets)

Mid-afternoon (3.30 p.m.)
(Supplement—drink)

Dinner (7.00 p.m.)
Red meat or poultry
Rice or baked potato
Vegetables
Tea or coffee
(Supplement—tablets)

Supper (9.30 p.m.)
Cold meat
Hard-boiled eggs
Cheese
Nuts
(Supplement—drink)

DIET TYPE B

Breakfast (7.00 a.m.)
3 or 4 bananas
Glass of non-fat milk
(Supplement—tablets)

Mid-morning (9.30 a.m.)
Fruit
(Supplement—drink)

Pre-workout (11.30 a.m.)
(Supplement—tablets)

Lunch (2.00 p.m.)
2 chicken breasts
Non-fat milk
Fruit until not hungry

Pre-workout (4.00 p.m.)
(Supplement—tablets)

Dinner (8.00 p.m.)
Chicken breasts
Vegetables (beans, peas,
  carrots, potatoes)
Pasta
Ice cream

Before Bed
(Supplement—Drink)

The supplements mentioned in the tables are of two kinds: tablets and drinks. Tablets will usually consist of various combinations of amino acids, vitamins and minerals, while drinks will again contain amino acids and sometimes digestive enzymes, fibre and/or vitamins, minerals and carbohydrates. If the supplements are taken with food, tablets are usually best taken 20 minutes before the meal and the protein drink at your leisure after the meal; however, it is best to follow any instructions given on the pack, ensuring (as stated above) that you do not exceed recommended dosages. The common factor is provided by the high content of amino acids, which are the key subunits of which the protein molecule chain is composed and are sometimes referred to as the 'building blocks' of protein. In all, there are twenty different amino acids which are linked and repeated in endless variations to form individual proteins. Commercial bodybuilding diet supplements are compounded from sources rich in protein, and their amino acid content (arginine, ornithine, lysine, etc.) will be listed on the packet or container.

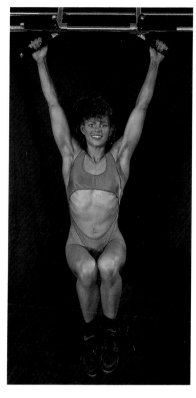

Gina Randall, Australian figure-form champion, demonstrates Matrix Hanging Leg Raises.

General nutritional advice

The extent to which trainers are able to follow a rigid dietary programme of the kind set out above will obviously vary from one individual to another—depending, for example, on one's hours of work and on family and other commitments; nonetheless, there are a number of general principles which almost all trainers will be able to apply to their eating habits in order to support and enhance the effectiveness of their weight programme.

Vary your protein sources

Weight trainers often develop the habit of eating exactly the same foods day after day, either because they assume this is the best way of monitoring their food intake, or simply because of convenience. Not only does this type of eating regime become boring, it is also likely to lead to deficiencies in the diet.

A diet which relied primarily on tuna and chicken for the daily protein intake, for example, could be considered deficient, since neither chicken nor fish has the amino acid balance required to be considered a 'perfect' protein source. Although sometimes considered a complete protein, chicken is low in some essential amino acids; namely some of the branched-chain amino acids which are important in building and maintaining muscle mass.

Eating from the same protein sources every day may lead to a deficiency in one or more amino acids: this may actually reduce muscle growth, since the body will be forced to sacrifice a muscle cell in order to access an essential amino acid. This is one reason why the use of supplements may be beneficial. As Brian Sharkey points out:

> More important than the quantity of protein in the diet is the quality, because certain amino acids cannot be synthesized in the body. Thus these *essential* amino acids must be provided in the diet. Failure to supply one of the essential amino acids will put a halt to the synthesis of proteins containing that building block.[2]

Deriving protein from a variety of sources such as turkey, lean pork, a variety of fish, different kinds of beans (especially brown beans), lean beef, tofu and lentils, in addition to a regular intake from well-known sources such as chicken breast and tuna, can help prevent deficiencies and ensure that full use is made of every gram of protein consumed.

The importance of timing

The aim of an appropriate nutritional programme will be to provide the body with its needs at the time when they are most required. The timing of the food intake thus needs to be carefully coordinated with the timing of the training programme; for example, some bodybuilders and other athletes trying to add to their muscle mass will attempt simply to maximise the amount of food they consume over a 24-hour period, and will consume a large meal (possibly accompanied by supplements) late at night or just before retiring. Such habits may favour the accumulation of several kilograms of fat, but late-night meals are quite ineffective as a means of favouring the growth of muscle.

The body's metabolic rate is highest during the morning and early afternoon hours. Most nutrients are digested, absorbed and utilised most efficiently at this time, which is thus the time of day at which the greatest number of kilojoules (or calories) should be taken in.

Large meals late at night, especially if they are high in protein, can also interfere with sleeping patterns: too much protein can increase the metabolic rate at the very time when the muscles should be engaged in the process of repair and recuperation. Excessive carbohydrates consumed late in the evening are more likely to be stored as fat than as glycogen because energy demands are lower.

It is best to allocate the food intake in such a way that the vast majority of kilojoules (at least 75 per cent) is taken in before evening. You can still have an evening snack, but preferably one that is a combination of carbohydrates and protein and is low in fat.

Cook with care

Depending on cooking and preparation methods, the nutrient content of foods can vary greatly. Some cooking procedures can significantly reduce vitamins and minerals and destroy proteins, thus removing much of the value of what might appear to be a nutritious dietary regime.

Freshness is important. Do not let foods sit around for long periods on the kitchen bench or even in the refrigerator. Try to avoid pre-cutting fruits or vegetables since this leads to dehydration and nutrient breakdown.

Do not overcook foods. Prolonged exposure to high temperatures destroys vitamins and protein—not to mention flavour. Cook vegetables until they soften slightly, but are still colourful and crisp. Steaming, stir-frying (with a minuscule amount of fat) and microwaving are best. If you boil vegetables, use a minimum of water to avoid burning or sticking, use preheated water and cover tightly. (Cruciferous vegetables like broccoli and cauliflower are the exception—they should remain uncovered to allow bitter-tasting sulphur to escape.)

Eat small, frequent meals

This is extremely important. Small, frequent meals are easier for your body to digest, absorb and assimilate. They help to keep your metabolic rate active and minimise the possibility that fat will be stored.

The mechanical, chemical and enzymatic processes involved in breaking foods down into components small enough to pass through the walls of the intestine are accomplished most efficiently with a smaller quantity of food.

Small meals also help stabilise blood levels of amino acids and sugar, which helps promote more constant energy levels and better appetite (since appetite is largely influenced by blood sugar levels). Consuming food frequently also minimises catabolic pathways since nutrients are supplied every few hours.

Chew thoroughly

This may appear self-evident, but chewing is the first and arguably the most important phase of food breakdown for digestion. The fact is that most of us eat much too fast and don't chew our food nearly well enough. Most of the mechanical breakdown of food is accomplished during chewing, which increases the surface area of the food so that digestive acids and enzymes can work efficiently. Chewing also mixes food with saliva, which contains amylase, the enzyme which initiates carbohydrate digestion.

Inadequate chewing allows large clumps of food to enter the digestive tract, reducing digestive efficiency, leading to indigestion, flatulence (gas) and bloating as intestinal bacteria have less time to digest food particles which should have been broken down earlier. This means less efficient absorption of the food and a decrease in nutrient absorption.

For these reasons, it is important to eat meals in as relaxed an atmosphere as possible, and especially to take small mouthfuls and chew food thoroughly before swallowing.

Drink the right thing at the right time

Most sedentary people should drink at least eight to ten 227 millilitre (8 ounce) glasses of water per day. Those who exercise should drink even more water, especially in warm environments or if they sweat profusely.

If you feel you should cut back on your intake of water because you are 'holding' water, you are in all likelihood mistaken. The less you drink, the greater the need (and the tendency) for the body to hold onto or retain its water content. (This does not apply to those bodybuilders who are preparing for a contest, and who may accustom their bodies over a period of ten days or so to a reduced water intake.)

While water is critical to fat metabolism, protein digestion and organ function, too much water with meals can interfere with nutrient digestion and absorption. We tend to eat too fast and drink too much water with our meals, especially if we feel both hungry and thirsty after training. This will dilute acids and enzymes in the digestive tract, and thus compromise digestion.

With meals, you should drink whatever moderate amount of water is necessary to enjoy the meal comfortably—say, a glass or two at most. If you come home thirsty from the gym, drink water straight away—before you eat. This water will be absorbed quickly and not lead to the problems mentioned above. Drink most of your water intake between meals throughout the day.

Carbonated soft drinks, whether diet or not, should be avoided with meals, especially protein meals. These drinks can drastically dilute and neutralise stomach acids essential for digestion.

Enjoy other beverages—including coffee, tea, etc.—in moderation as they may cause the body to excrete minerals such as sodium, potassium or calcium. Many trainers find it helpful to substitute a protein drink for their mealtime cup of tea or coffee, usually in a less concentrated form than for their between-meal 'snack'.

Eat natural foods

You should avoid processed and refined foods whenever possible. Such foods are typically high in added fat, sugar and sodium, but they also have had many of their vitamins and minerals stripped from them.

It is sensible to make a habit of reading the labels on packaged food noting, in particular, the volume of artificial additives present. High-temperature processing can also be detrimental to nutritional content.

If pressure of time, family preference or other factors result in your eating relatively large amounts of processed or convenience foods, your diet may lack adequate supplies of vitamins and minerals. Those people—especially weight trainers—who come into this category can help redress their dietary imbalance by taking multivitamin tablets regularly.

Consume fresh fruits, vegetables and juices

Raw fruit and raw vegetables can serve as an excellent snack. Vegetable and fruit juices are preferable to soft drinks, especially if they can be juiced or blended at home for immediate consumption.

Fresh fruit juices contain active enzymes that would be destroyed rapidly if they were processed. The same is true of canned vegetables which are processed at high temperatures: food processing can decrease the chromium content of foods by as much as 80 per cent; other vitamin and mineral contents are known to suffer as well. Freshly squeezed and bottled juices, however, retain their nutritional value; read the bottle label carefully to check for vitamin and mineral content.

Finally, do not try to rush things. 'Crash' weight-reduction or weight-gain programmes should be avoided in favour of longer-term dietary (and, where relevant, supplementation) regimes to which the body can accustom itself. It is true that excessive protein ingestion has no harmful effect provided that the diet includes an appropriate balance of carbohydrate and fat, but the excess protein will not be stored in the body: the nitrogen molecules will simply be stripped and eliminated through the urine, while the remaining carbon skeleton will be converted to glucose or fat. The overall aim should therefore be to match diet and supplementation as closely as possible to the demands of the training regime: the more vigorous the latter, the greater the need for protein and the higher the rate of contractile protein synthesis. Thus, as you progress in your Matrix training from one level of muscular challenge to the next, the more effectively your attention to an appropriate and sustaining diet will contribute to muscle growth. The exceptional intensity of Matrix training maximises the body's need for increased protein uptake in response to energy expenditure, which means that a higher proportion of ingested protein is directed to muscle growth than is the case with less demanding regimes.

As reported in the Matrix supplementation trials, the greatest overall degree of muscle gain occurred in those subjects who had used a combination of Matrix training and protein supplementation. Whilst it may be concluded from these results that the use of supplements enhanced the training effect, it seems equally possible, in the light of the above, that the intense demands of Matrix training assisted in optimising the hypertrophic effect of the supplements themselves. Confirmation of this hypothesis must await the outcome of further trials currently being conducted.

References

1   The commercial supplements used in the controlled tests were the Weider 'Victory' range of supplements.
2   Sharkey, *Physiology of Fitness*, p. 131.

4   The training programme

The Matrix routines set out in this chapter are organised into four separate twelve-week programmes, making a total of 48 weeks or virtually a full year's training. Each programme consists of:

- Core routines for the major body parts (i.e. chest, thighs, shoulders, lats and back, biceps and triceps);
- areas of specialisation such as calves, forearms and abdominals, any or all of which can be incorporated as desired into the four twelve-week core programmes. (Detailed routines are given in chapter 6)
  Each of the four programmes is complete and self-contained, and it is strongly recommended that each be fully mastered before you move onto the programme following.

Achieving goals

Important: Only very advanced trainers will be able to complete the four programmes within a year, using the weekly training schedule provided in chapter 2 of this book. Unless you are a very advanced trainer, you should note carefully the following advice:

- Do not attempt to rush through the whole of the four programmes within a year, just so that you can say that you have completed them in that time. As we stated in chapter 2, you will only be cheating yourself;
- The idea is to complete the programmes using strict form and the short pauses indicated in the instructions; depending on your age, sex, physical fitness and other factors, it may take you two, three or even more years to complete the entire course. You may, for instance, need not twelve, but 24 or more weeks to complete the first programme, before moving onto the second;
- Each of the four programmes should be completed before you move onto the next; that is, you should be able to perform the routine exactly as set out—with the pauses specified and without sacrificing form. If, for

43

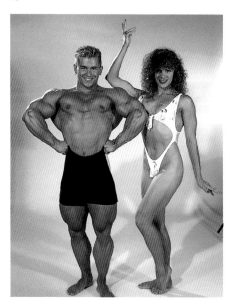

World champion Lee Priest and Gina
Randall.

example, in the shoulder routine you are swaying your back, pressing the
weight up unevenly or using your legs to push the bar up, you are not
using correct form and the weight is too heavy.

Less advanced trainers, or those who are new to Matrix training, should
therefore begin by treating the prescribed routines as a guide to what they
are aiming to achieve by the time they complete the programme—not as a
prescription for what they must achieve in the early stages of training.

In any routine, simply do the best you can using your maximum effort.
Do not 'go easy on yourself'—Matrix training needs to be intense and
demanding in order to be effective—but at the same time, do not leave
yourself totally exhausted so that your recuperation suffers and you are still
tired by your next training session.

To help accustom yourself to the demands of Matrix training, you can:

- Increase the pauses between sets. Try doubling the pause-time specified,
  then cutting it back by five seconds each week until you reach the
  pause-time given in the instructions;
- Decrease the weight. Drop the weight you have been using by 2.5 kg (or
  5 lb) or even 5 kg (or 10 lb) until you reach a weight that is light enough
  to let you complete the required repetition pattern;
- Break up the sets. As well as the pauses between sets, you can pause
  briefly within a set; as little as five seconds will sometimes enable you
  to recuperate sufficiently to complete the required set before passing on
  to the next.

Once you have progressively grown accustomed to this form of training,
you will be able to perform the routines as specified. **This is your goal,
however long it takes you to reach it.**

When you can perform all the routines in Programme I exactly as set out in the instructions, you are ready to move onto Programme II, and so on.

Each programme is more difficult than the programme preceding. This is achieved by the progressive addition of more demanding Matrix techniques from one programme to the next. The four programmes set out here gradually shift the emphasis from the twelve basic Matrix techniques to a further twelve techniques (known as Intermediate routines) which are designed to 'blitz' the target muscles by pushing them to increasingly difficult levels of diversity and cumulative overload.

The Matrix training techniques

The twelve basic techniques are as follows:

1 Conventional Matrix
2 Descending Matrix
3 Ascending Matrix
4 Matrix alternates
5 Cumulative Matrix alternates
6 Matrix ladders
7 Cumulative Matrix ladders
8 Ascending iso-Matrix
9 Descending iso-Matrix
10 Conventional iso-Matrix
11 Cumulative iso-Matrix
12 Mixed iso-Matrix

To these are added the following twelve intermediate techniques:

1 Matrix steps
2 Matrix giant steps
3 Iso-Matrix steps
4 Cumulative iso-Matrix steps
5 Iso-Matrix giant steps
6 Matrix reversals
7 Descending Matrix reversals
8 Ascending Matrix reversals
9 Cumulative Matrix reversals
10 Matrix composites
11 Matrix reverse ladders
12 Matrix reverse step ladders

As you progress through the four programmes, your workout schedule will contain more and more of the intermediate techniques woven in with the basic techniques, to provide a total programme designed for maximum muscle growth.

The 24 techniques used in this book are set out in the tables below. It is a good idea to spend some time studying them. Concentrate particularly on the diagrams which accompany the instructions, so that you can discern the *pattern* of movements which each of them involves. The techniques are not as hard to remember as may at first seem, and as you become more and more familiar with the pattern of movements underlying each of them you will be able to free yourself progressively from constant reference to the text as you perform the Matrix routines.

The diagrams show each repetition as a column, the length of the column representing either a full or a part-repetition. You will note that half-up and half-down reps are shown as slightly longer than a half column, a reminder that you should bring the weight just slightly further than the half-way position on half-up and half-down movements. In the iso-Matrix techniques, some of the columns contain a number of dots: these correspond to the number of seconds for which you should hold the weight at the position specified. Thus, a 'half-up' column containing three dots represents a movement which is held at the half-up position for three seconds, and so on.

1 Conventional Matrix

5 full reps
5 half-up
5 half-down
5 full reps

2 Descending Matrix

7 full reps
6 half-up
5 half-down
4 full reps

3 Ascending Matrix

4 full reps
5 half-up
6 half-down
7 full reps

4 Matrix Alternates

5 full reps
  +
1 half-up
1 half-down
1 full rep   +
  +
1 half-up
1 half-down
2 full reps

1 half-up
1 half-down
3 full reps
  +
1 half-up
1 half-down
4 full reps
  +
1 half-up
1 half-down
5 full reps

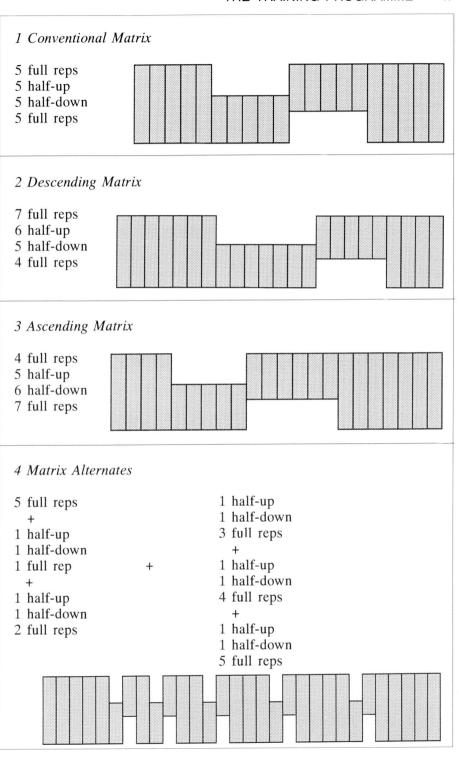

5 *Cumulative Matrix Alternates*

1 full rep	3 half-up
1 half-up	3 half-down
1 half-down	4 full reps
2 full reps	+
+ +	4 half-up
2 half-up	4 half-down
2 half-down	5 full reps
3 full reps	

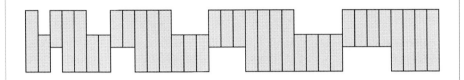

6 *Matrix Ladders*

5 full reps	1 rep 1/5 down
+	1 rep 2/5 down
1 rep 1/5 up	1 rep 3/5 down
1 rep 2/5 up +	1 rep 4/5 down
1 rep 3/5 up	1 full rep
1 rep 4/5 up	+
+	5 full reps
1 full rep	

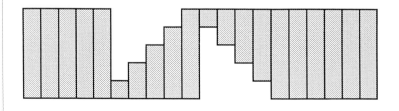

7 *Cumulative Matrix Ladders*

1 full rep
+
1 rep 1/5 up
2 reps 2/5 up
3 reps 3/5 up   +
4 reps 4/5 up
+
5 full reps

1 rep 1/5 down
2 reps 2/5 down
3 reps 3/5 down
4 reps 4/5 down
+
5 full reps

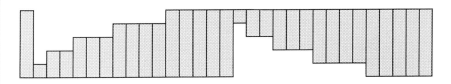

8 *Ascending iso-Matrix*

5 full reps
+
1 half-up (holding weight in the half position for 1 second)
1 half-up (hold for 2 seconds)
1 half-up (hold for 3 seconds)
1 half-up (hold for 4 seconds)
1 half-up (hold for 5 seconds)
1 full rep
+
1 half-down (holding weight in the half position for 1 second)
1 half-down (hold for 2 seconds)
1 half-down (hold for 3 seconds)
1 half-down (hold for 4 seconds)
1 half-down (hold for 5 seconds)
+
5 full reps

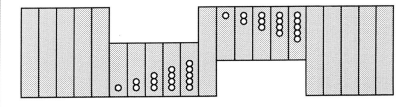

9 Descending iso-Matrix

5 full reps
+
1 half-up (holding weight in the half position for 5 seconds)
1 half-up (hold for 4 seconds)
1 half-up (hold for 3 seconds)
1 half-up (hold for 2 seconds)
1 half-up (hold for 1 second)
+
1 full rep
+
1 half-down (holding weight in the half position for 5 seconds)
1 half-down (hold for 4 seconds)
1 half-down (hold for 3 seconds)
1 half-down (hold for 2 seconds)
1 half-down (hold for 1 second)
+
5 full reps

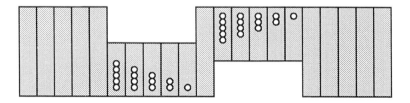

10 Conventional iso-Matrix

5 full reps
+
5 half-up (hold for 5 seconds)
5 half-down (hold for 5 seconds)
+
5 full reps

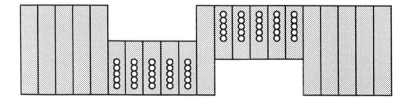

11 Cumulative iso-Matrix

1 full rep
+
1 half-up (hold for 1 second)
2 half-up (hold each rep for 2 seconds)
3 half-up (hold each rep for 3 seconds)
4 half-up (hold each rep for 4 seconds)
+
5 full reps
+
1 half-down (hold for 1 second)
2 half-down (hold each rep for 2 seconds)
3 half-down (hold each rep for 3 seconds)
4 half-down (hold each rep for 4 seconds)
+
5 full reps

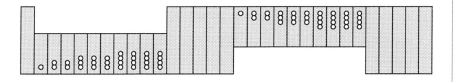

12 Mixed iso-Matrix

5 full reps
+
3 half-up (hold each for 3 seconds)
3 half-down (no holding)
3 half-up (no holding)
3 half-down (hold each rep for 3 seconds)
+
5 full reps

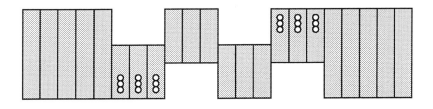

13 Matrix Steps

5 full reps
  +
1 half-up
2 half-down
3 half-up
4 half-down
5 half-up
6 half-down
  +
5 full reps

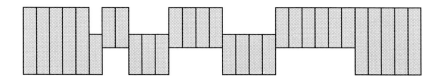

14 Matrix Giant Steps

5 full reps
  +
1 half-up
2 half-down
  +
3 full reps
  +
4 half-up
5 half-down
  +
6 full reps

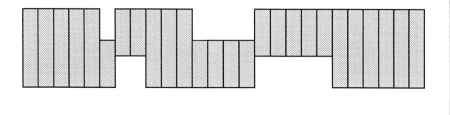

15 Isomatrix Steps

1 full rep
+
2 half-up (hold each rep for 3 seconds)
3 half-down (hold each rep for 3 seconds)
4 half-up (hold each rep for 3 seconds)
5 half-down (hold each rep for 3 seconds)
+
6 full reps

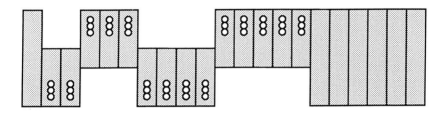

16 Cumulative Isomatrix Steps

1 full rep
+
2 half-up (hold each rep for 3 seconds)
3 half-down (hold each rep for 4 seconds)
4 half-up (hold each rep for 5 seconds)
5 half-down (hold each rep for 6 seconds)
+
6 full reps

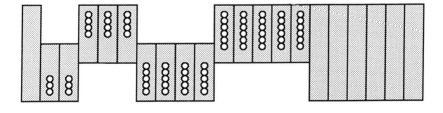

17 Isomatrix Giant Steps

5 full reps
    +
1 half-up (hold for 5 seconds)
2 half-down (hold each rep for 4 seconds)
    +
3 full reps
    +
4 half-up (hold each rep for 3 seconds)
5 half-down (hold each rep for 2 seconds)
    +
6 full reps

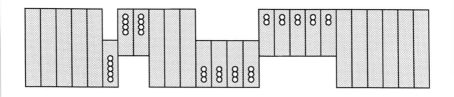

18 Matrix Reversals

5 full reps
    +
1 rep 3/4 up
1 rep 3/4 down
    +
1 rep 3/4 up
1 rep 3/4 down
    +
1 rep 3/4 up
1 rep 3/4 down
    +
5 full reps

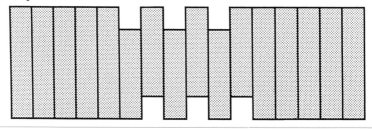

19 Descending Matrix Reversals

7 full reps
  +
1 rep 3/4 up
1 rep 3/4 down
  +
6 full reps
  +
1 rep 3/4 up
1 rep 3/4 down
  +
5 full reps

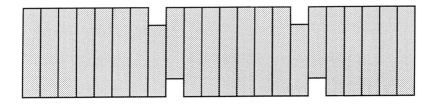

20 Ascending Matrix Reversals

5 full reps
  +
1 rep 3/4 up
1 rep 3/4 down
  +
6 full reps
    +
1 rep 3/4 up
1 rep 3/4 down
  +
7 full reps

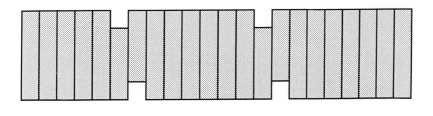

21 *Cumulative Matrix Reversals*

3 full reps
+
3 reps 3/4 up
3 reps 3/4 down
+
4 full reps
+
4 reps 3/4 up
4 reps 3/4 down
+
5 full reps

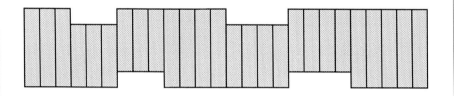

22 *Matrix Composites*

5 full reps
+
3 half-up
3 half-down
+
3 half-up
3 half-down
+
3 half-up
3 half-down
+
5 full reps

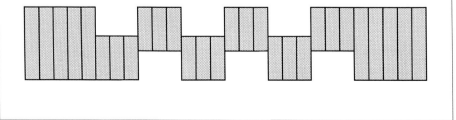

23 Matrix Reverse Ladders

5 full reps
+
1 rep 1/5 up
1 rep 1/5 down
+
1 rep 2/5 up
1 rep 2/5 down
+
1 rep 3/5 up
1 rep 3/5 down
+
1 rep 4/5 up
1 rep 4/5 down
+
5 full reps

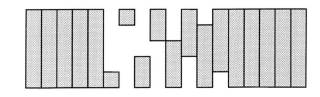

24 Matrix Reverse Step Ladders

1 full rep
+
2 reps 1/5 up
3 reps 1/5 down
+
4 reps 2/5 up
5 reps 2/5 down
+
6 reps 3/5 up
7 reps 3/5 down
+
8 reps 4/5 up
9 reps 4/5 down
+
1 full rep

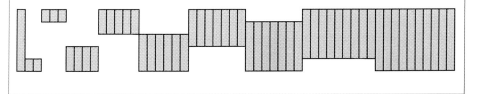

Note on performing part-movements: For *half-up* movements, the weight should be raised to just above the half-way point of the movement. For *half-down* movements, the weight should be lowered to just below the half-way point of the movement. When a series of part reps is followed by full reps, ensure that you *complete* the part reps first. For example, at the end of a series of half-down bench presses followed by full presses, you should return the bar to the fully extended position on completion of the last half-down rep before lowering it to the chest to begin the full reps. When a part rep in one direction is followed by a part rep in the other direction, ensure that you complete the first rep before moving on to the second. This occurs, for example, in Matrix Reversals (including Ascending and Descending Reversals), when a rep 3/4 up is followed immediately by a rep 3/4 down. If performing barbell curls, you would raise the bar to the 3/4 up position, then fully lower it to complete the rep; you would then raise the bar to the up position (the starting point for the next movement), lower it to the 3/4 down position and return to the starting point (the up position) to complete the rep. When the instruction is to 'hold for 5 seconds', the intention is that the bar or dumbbells will be held stationary at one or other of the half position or fractional positions for the time specified.

PART II

The Matrix System
in practice

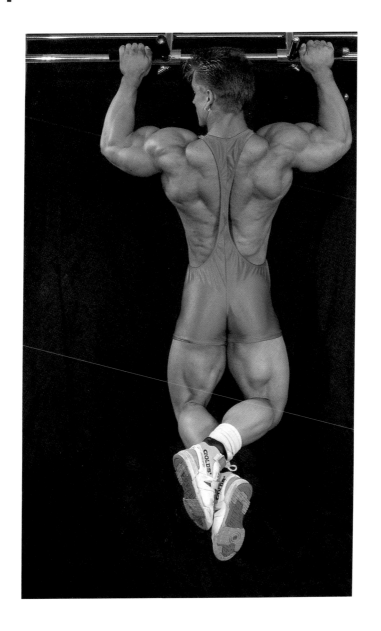

5 Matrix core routines

I Matrix core routines: weeks 1–12

Chest Matrix

Stage 1

Sequence A

(a) *Matrix Steps Bench Press*
    5 full reps
       +
    1 half-up
    2 half-down
    3 half-up
    4 half-down
    5 half-up
    6 half-down
       +
    5 full reps

    20 seconds pause

(b) *Conventional Matrix Bench Press*
    5 full reps
    5 half-up
    5 half-down
    5 full reps

    25 seconds pause

(c) *Matrix Giant Steps Bench Press*
   5 full reps
      +
   1 half-up
   2 half-down
      +
   3 full reps
      +
   4 half-up
   5 half-down
      +
   6 full reps

   30 seconds pause

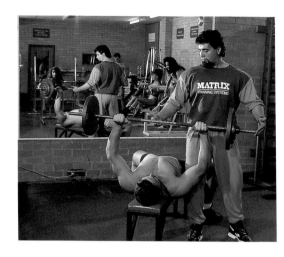

Matrix Giant Steps Bench Press

(d) *Descending Matrix Incline Press*
   7 full reps
   6 half-up
   5 half-down
   4 full reps

   40 seconds pause

(e) *Matrix Steps Pec Deck*
   5 full reps
      +
   1 half-up
   2 half-down
   3 half-up
   4 half-down
   5 half-up
   6 half-down
      +
   5 full reps

   25 seconds pause

(f) *Conventional iso-Matrix Pec Deck*
   5 full reps
      +
   5 half-up (hold for 3 seconds*)
   5 half-down (hold for 3 seconds)
      +
   5 full reps

   2 minutes pause

Sequence B

(a) *Iso-Matrix Steps Bench Press*
   1 full rep
      +
   2 half-up (hold each rep for 3 seconds)
   3 half-down (hold each rep for 3 seconds)
   4 half-up (hold each rep for 3 seconds)
   5 half-down (hold each rep for 3 seconds)
      +
   6 full reps

   20 seconds pause

(b) *Ascending Matrix Bench Press*
   4 full reps
   5 half-up
   6 half-down
   7 full reps

   25 seconds pause

(c) *Matrix Giant Steps Dumbbell Flyes*
   5 full reps
      +
   1 half-up
   2 half-down
      +
   3 full reps
      +
   4 half-up
   5 half-down
      +
   6 full reps

   30 seconds pause

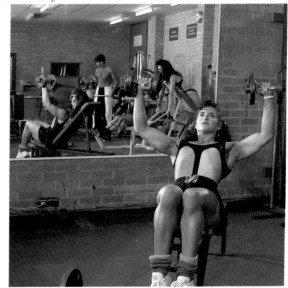

Matrix Giant Steps Dumbbell
Flyes

(d) *Conventional Matrix Dumbbell Flyes*
   5 full reps
   5 half-up
   5 half-down
   5 full reps

   Finish

Thigh Matrix

Stage 1

Sequence A

(a) *Matrix Giant Steps Leg Press*
    5 full reps
    +
    1 half-up
    2 half-down
    +
    3 full reps
    +
    4 half-up
    5 half-down
    +
    6 full reps

    20 seconds pause

(b) *Ascending Matrix Leg Press*
    4 full reps
    5 half-up
    6 half-down
    7 full reps

    25 seconds pause

(c) *Matrix Alternates Leg Press*

5 full reps		1 half-up
+		1 half-down
1 half-up		3 full reps
1 half-down		+
1 full rep	+	1 half-up
+		1 half-down
1 half-up		4 full reps
1 half-down		+
2 full reps		1 half-up
		1 half-down
		5 full reps

    50 seconds pause

(d) *Iso-Matrix Steps Leg Press*
   1 full rep
      +
   2 half-up (hold each rep for 3 seconds)
   3 half-down (hold each rep for 3 seconds)
   4 half-up (hold each rep for 3 seconds)
   5 half-down (hold each rep for 3 seconds)
      +
   6 full reps

   50 seconds pause

(e) *Matrix Steps Leg Extensions*
   5 full reps
      +
   1 half-up
   2 half-down
   3 half-up
   4 half-down
   5 half-up
   6 half-down
      +
   5 full reps

   20 seconds pause

(f) *Cumulative iso-Matrix Steps Leg Extensions*
   1 full rep
      +
   2 half-up (hold each rep for 3 seconds)
   3 half-down (hold each rep for 4 seconds)
   4 half-up (hold each rep for 5 seconds)
   5 half-down (hold each rep for 6 seconds)
      +
   6 full reps

   2 minutes pause

Sequence B

(a) *Matrix Giant Steps Leg Extensions*
    5 full reps
      +
    1 half-up
    2 half-down
      +
    3 full reps
      +
    4 half-up
    5 half-down
      +
    6 full reps
    30 seconds pause

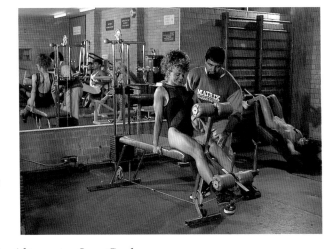

Matrix Giant Steps Leg
Extensions

(b) *Cumulative Matrix Alternates Leg Curls*

1 full rep	3 half-up
1 half-up	3 half-down
1 half-down	4 full reps
2 full reps +	+
+	4 half-up
2 half-up	4 half-down
2 half-down	5 full reps
3 full reps	

    40 seconds pause

(c) *Iso-Matrix Steps Leg Curls*
    1 full rep
      +
    2 half-up (hold each rep for 3 seconds)
    3 half-down (hold each rep for 3 seconds)
    4 half-up (hold each rep for 3 seconds)
    5 half-down (hold each rep for 3 seconds)
      +
    6 full reps
    30 seconds pause

(d) *Descending Matrix Leg Curls*
    7 full reps
    6 half-up
    5 half-down
    4 full reps
    Finish

Biceps Matrix

Stage 1

Sequence A

(a) *Matrix Steps Standing Barbell Curls*
  5 full reps
     +
  1 half-up
  2 half-down
  3 half-up
  4 half-down
  5 half-up
  6 half-down
     +
  5 full reps

  20 seconds pause

(b) *Conventional Matrix Standing Barbell Curls*
  5 full reps
  5 half-up
  5 half-down
  5 full reps

  30 seconds pause

(c) *Matrix Giant Steps Standing Barbell Curls*
  5 full reps
     +
  1 half-up
  2 half-down
     +
  3 full reps
     +
  4 half-up
  5 half-down
     +
  6 full reps

  40 seconds pause

(d) *Iso-Matrix Steps Preacher Bench Curls*
1 full rep
+
2 half-up (hold each rep for 3 seconds)
3 half-down (hold each rep for 3 seconds)
4 half-up (hold each rep for 3 seconds)
5 half-down (hold each rep for 3 seconds)
+
6 full reps

40 seconds pause

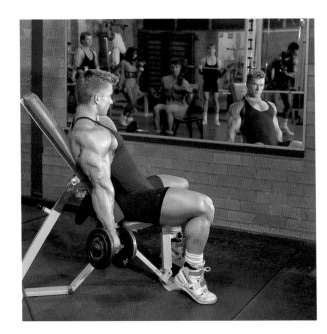

Lee Priest in the starting position for Matrix Incline Bench Dumbbell Curls.

(e) *Matrix Ladder Preacher Bench Curls*

5 full reps	1 rep 1/5 down
+	1 rep 2/5 down
1 rep 1/5 up	1 rep 3/5 down
1 rep 2/5 up +	1 rep 4/5 down
1 rep 3/5 up	1 full rep
1 rep 4/5 up	+
+	5 full reps
1 full rep	

Pause 3 minutes

Sequence B

(a) *Matrix Giant Steps Incline Bench Dumbbell Curls*
5 full reps
+
1 half-up
2 half-down
+
3 full reps
+
4 half-up
5 half-down
+
6 full reps

40 seconds pause

(b) *Descending Matrix Incline Bench Dumbbell Curls*
7 full reps
6 half-up
5 half-down
4 full reps

30 seconds pause

(c) *Cumulative Matrix Ladders Incline Bench Dumbbell Curls*

1 full rep	1 rep 1/5 down
+	2 reps 2/5 down
1 rep 1/5 up	3 reps 3/5 down
2 reps 2/5 up	4 reps 4/5 down
3 reps 3/5 up +	+
4 reps 4/5 up	5 full reps
+	
5 full reps	

40 seconds pause

(d) *Cumulative Iso-Matrix Steps Preacher Bench Curls*
1 full rep
+
2 half-up (hold each rep for 3 seconds)
3 half-down (hold each rep for 4 seconds)
4 half-up (hold each rep for 5 seconds)
5 half-down (hold each rep for 6 seconds)
+
6 full reps

Finish

Triceps Matrix

Stage 1

Sequence A

(a) *Conventional Matrix Lying Triceps Press*
       5 full reps
       5 half-up
       5 half-down
       5 full reps

       20 seconds pause

(b) *Matrix Steps Lying Triceps Press*
       5 full reps
          +
       1 half-up
       2 half-down
       3 half-up
       4 half-down
       5 half-up
       6 half-down
          +
       5 full reps

       25 seconds pause

(c) *Matrix Giant Steps Triceps Pushdowns*
       5 full reps
          +
       1 half-up
       2 half-down
          +
       3 full reps
          +
       4 half-up
       5 half-down
          +
       6 full reps

       30 seconds pause

(d) *Iso-matrix Steps Triceps Pushdowns*
   1 full rep
   +
   2 half-up (hold each rep for 3 seconds)
   3 half-down (hold each rep for 3 seconds)
   4 half-up (hold each rep for 3 seconds)
   5 half-down (hold each rep for 3 seconds)
   +
   6 full reps

   40 seconds pause

(e) *Matrix Alternates Lying Triceps Press*

5 full reps	1 half-up
+	1 half-down
1 half-up	3 full reps
1 half-down +	+
1 full rep	1 half-up
+	1 half-down
1 half-up	4 full reps
1 half-down	+
2 full reps	1 half-up
	1 half-down
	5 full reps

   50 seconds pause

(f) *Ascending Matrix Lying Triceps Press*
   4 full reps
   5 half-up
   6 half-down
   7 full reps

   40 seconds pause

(g) *Cumulative Iso-Matrix Steps Triceps Pushdowns*
1 full rep
   +
1 half-up (hold for 1 second)
2 half-up (hold each rep for 2 seconds)
3 half-up (hold each rep for 3 seconds)
4 half-up (hold each rep for 4 seconds)
   +
5 full reps
   +
1 half-down (hold for 1 second)
2 half-down (hold each rep for 2 seconds)
3 half-down (hold each rep for 3 seconds)
4 half-down (hold each rep for 4 seconds)
   +
5 full reps

3 minutes pause

Sequence B

(a) *Matrix Steps Standing Overhead Triceps Press*
5 full reps
   +
1 half-up
2 half-down
3 half-up
4 half-down
5 half-up
6 half-down
   +
5 full reps

20 seconds pause

(b) *Descending Matrix Standing Overhead Triceps Press*
7 full reps
6 half-up
5 half-down
4 full reps

25 seconds pause

(c) *Matrix Giant Steps Lying Triceps Press*
5 full reps
+
1 half-up
2 half-down
+
3 full. reps
+
4 half-up
5 half-down
+
6 full reps

30 seconds pause

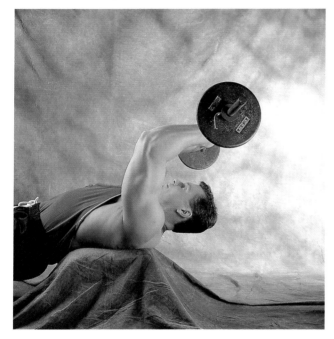

Australian heavy-weight
champion Paul Haslam
demonstrating Matrix
Lying Triceps Press.

(d) *Iso-matrix Steps Standing Overhead Triceps Press*
1 full rep
+
2 half-up (hold each rep for 3 seconds)
3 half-down (hold each rep for 3 seconds)
4 half-up (hold each rep for 3 seconds)
5 half-down (hold each rep for 3 seconds)
+
6 full reps

Finish

Deltoid Matrix

Stage 1

Sequence A

(a) *Matrix Roll Press*
   15 full reps

   20 seconds pause

(b) *Matrix Steps Press Behind the Neck*
   5 full reps
     +
   1 half-up
   2 half-down
   3 half-up
   4 half-down
   5 half-up
   6 half-down
     +
   5 full reps

   25 seconds pause

(c) *Matrix Giant Steps Press in Front of the Neck*
   5 full reps
     +
   1 half-up
   2 half-down
     +
   3 full reps
     +
   4 half-up
   5 half-down
     +
   6 full reps

   30 seconds pause

(d) *Matrix Roll Press*
   15 full reps

   25 seconds pause

(e) *Matrix Alternates Dumbbell Lateral Raises*

5 full reps	1 half-up
+	1 half-down
1 half-up	3 full reps
1 half-down +	+
1 full rep	1 half-up
+	1 half-down
1 half-up	4 full reps
1 half-down	+
2 full reps	1 half-up
	1 half-down
	5 full reps

20 seconds pause

(f) *Iso-Matrix Steps Dumbbell Front Raises*
1 full rep
    +
2 half-up (hold each rep for 3 seconds)
3 half-down (hold each rep for 3 seconds)
4 half-up (hold each rep for 3 seconds)
5 half-down (hold each rep for 3 seconds)
    +
6 full reps

2 minutes pause

Sequence B

(a) *Matrix Roll Press*
15 full reps

20 seconds pause

(b) *Cumulative Matrix Alternates Press Behind the Neck*

1 full rep	3 half-up
1 half-up	3 half-down
1 half-down	4 full reps
2 full reps +	+
+	4 half-up
2 half-up	4 half-down
2 half-down	5 full reps
3 full reps	

25 seconds pause

(c) *Cumulative Iso-Matrix Steps Press in Front of the Neck*
    1 full rep
       +
    2 half-up (hold each rep for 3 seconds)
    3 half-down (hold each rep for 4 seconds)
    4 half-up (hold each rep for 5 seconds)
    5 half-down (hold each rep for 6 seconds)
       +
    6 full reps

    40 seconds pause

(d) *Matrix Roll Press*
    15 full reps

    25 seconds pause

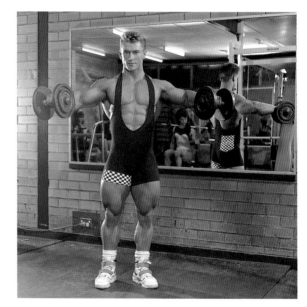

Matrix Steps Dumbbell Lateral
Raises

(e) *Matrix Steps Dumbbell Lateral Raises*
    5 full reps
       +
    1 half-up
    2 half-down
    3 half-up
    4 half-down
    5 half-up
    6 half-down
       +
    5 full reps

    30 seconds pause

(f) *Matrix Ladders Dumbbell Front Raises*

5 full reps		1 rep 1/5 down
+		1 rep 2/5 down
1 rep 1/5 up		1 rep 3/5 down
1 rep 2/5 up	+	1 rep 4/5 down
1 rep 3/5 up		1 full rep
1 rep 4/5 up		+
+		5 full reps
1 full rep		

Finish

Lats and Back Matrix

Stage 1

Sequence A

(a) *Matrix Steps Bent-Over Rows*
   5 full reps
      +
   1 half-up
   2 half-down
   3 half-up
   4 half-down
   5 half-up
   6 half-down
      +
   5 full reps

   20 seconds pause

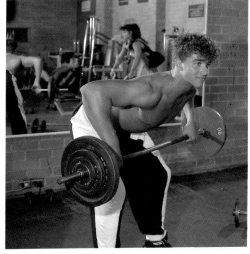

Matrix Steps Bent-Over Rows

(b) *Matrix Steps Lat Machine Pulldowns*
5 full reps
   +
1 half-up
2 half-down
3 half-up
4 half-down
5 half-up
6 half-down
   +
5 full reps

25 seconds pause

(c) *Matrix Giant Steps Bent-Over Rows*
5 full reps
   +
1 half-up
2 half-down
   +
3 full reps
   +
4 half-up
5 half-down
   +
6 full reps

35 seconds pause

(d) *Matrix Giant Steps Lat Machine Pulldowns*
5 full reps
   +
1 half-up
2 half-down
   +
3 full reps
   +
4 half-up
5 half-down
   +
6 full reps

45 seconds pause

(e) *Iso-Matrix Steps Lat Machine Pulldowns*
    1 full rep
       +
    2 half-up (hold each rep for 3 seconds)
    3 half-down (hold each rep for 3 seconds)
    4 half-up (hold each rep for 3 seconds)
    5 half-down (hold each rep for 3 seconds)
       +
    6 full reps

    30 seconds pause

(f) *Cumulative Iso-Matrix Steps Bent-Over Rows*
    1 full rep
       +
    2 half-up (hold each rep for 3 seconds)
    3 half-down (hold each rep for 4 seconds)
    4 half-up (hold each rep for 5 seconds)
    5 half-down (hold each rep for 6 seconds)
       +
    6 full reps

    3 minutes pause

Sequence B

(a) *Matrix Steps Hyperextensions*
    5 full reps
       +
    1 half-up
    2 half-down
    3 half-up
    4 half-down
    5 half-up
    6 half-down
       +
    5 full reps

    20 seconds pause

(b) *Matrix Alternates Hyperextensions*

5 full reps	1 half-up
+	1 half-down
1 half-up	3 full reps
1 half-down +	+
1 full rep	1 half-up
+	1 half-down
1 half-up	4 full reps
1 half-down	+
+	1 half-up
2 full reps	1 half-down
	5 full reps

20 seconds pause

(c) *Iso-Matrix Steps Hyperextensions*
1 full rep
+
2 half-up (hold each rep for 3 seconds)
3 half-down (hold each rep for 3 seconds)
4 half-up (hold each rep for 3 seconds)
5 half-down (hold each rep for 3 seconds)
+
6 full reps

20 seconds pause

(d) *Conventional Matrix Stiff-Legged Deadlifts*
5 full reps
5 half-up
5 half-down
5 full reps

20 seconds pause

(e) *Matrix Ladders Bent-Over Rows*

5 full reps	1 rep 1/5 down
+	1 rep 2/5 down
1 rep 1/5 up	1 rep 3/5 down
1 rep 2/5 up +	1 rep 4/5 down
1 rep 3/5 up	1 full rep
1 rep 4/5 up	+
	5 full reps
1 full rep	

Finish

II Matrix core routines: weeks 13–24

Chest Matrix

Stage 2

Sequence A

(a) *Iso-Matrix Giant Steps Bench Press*
    5 full reps
    +
    1 half-up (hold for 5 seconds)
    2 half-down (hold each rep for 4 seconds)
    +
    3 full reps
    +
    4 half-up (hold each rep for 3 seconds)
    5 half-down (hold each rep for 2 seconds)
    +
    6 full reps

    15 seconds pause

(b) *Matrix Reversals Decline Bench Press*
    5 full reps
    +
    1 rep 3/4 up
    1 rep 3/4 down
    +
    1 rep 3/4 up
    1 rep 3/4 down
    +
    1 rep 3/4 up
    1 rep 3/4 down
    +
    5 full reps

    20 seconds pause

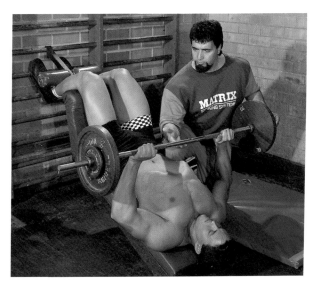

Matrix Reversals Decline Bench Press

(c) *Cumulative Matrix Ladders Bench Press*

1 full rep	1 rep 1/5 down
+	2 reps 2/5 down
1 rep 1/5 up	3 reps 3/5 down
2 reps 2/5 up	4 reps 4/5 down
3 reps 3/5 up +	+
4 reps 4/5 up	5 full reps
+	
5 full reps	

25 seconds pause

(d) *Ascending Iso-Matrix Bench Press*

5 full reps
+
1 half-up (holding weight in the half position for 1 second)
1 half-up (hold for 2 seconds)
1 half-up (hold for 3 seconds)
1 half-up (hold for 4 seconds)
1 half-up (hold for 5 seconds)
1 full rep
+
1 half-down (holding weight in the half position for 1 second)
1 half-down (hold for 2 seconds)
1 half-down (hold for 3 seconds)
1 half-down (hold for 4 seconds)
1 half-down (hold for 5 seconds)
+
5 full reps

30 seconds pause

(e) *Matrix Steps Incline Bench Press*

5 full reps
+
1 half-up
2 half-down
3 half-up
4 half-down
5 half-up
6 half-down
+
5 full reps

25 seconds pause

(f) *Iso-Matrix Steps Incline Bench Press*
1 full rep
+
2 half-up (hold each rep for 3 seconds)
3 half-down (hold each rep for 3 seconds)
4 half-up (hold each rep for 3 seconds)
5 half-down (hold each rep for 3 seconds)
+
6 full reps

20 seconds pause

(g) *Matrix Reversals Incline Bench Press*
5 full reps
+
1 rep 3/4 up
1 rep 3/4 down
+
1 rep 3/4 up
1 rep 3/4 down
+
1 rep 3/4 up
1 rep 3/4 down
+
5 full reps

2 minutes pause

Sequence B

(a) *Matrix Steps Dumbbell Flyes*
5 full reps
+
1 half-up
2 half-down
3 half-up
4 half-down
5 half-up
6 half-down
+
5 full reps

15 seconds pause

(b) *Iso-Matrix Giant Steps Pec Deck*
  5 full reps
  +
  1 half-up (hold for 5 seconds)
  2 half-down (hold each rep for 4 seconds)
  +
  3 full reps
  +
  4 half-up (hold each rep for 3 seconds)
  5 half-down (hold each rep for 2 seconds)
  +
  6 full reps

  15 seconds pause

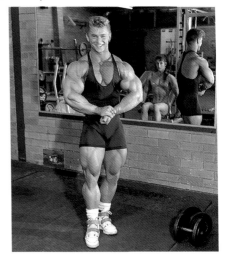

Lee Priest shows off his superb chest
development.

(c) *Descending Iso-Matrix Pec Deck*
  5 full reps
  +
  1 half-up (holding weight in the half position for 5 seconds)
  1 half-up (hold for 4 seconds)
  1 half-up (hold for 3 seconds)
  1 half-up (hold for 2 seconds)
  1 half-up (hold for 1 second)
  +
  1 full rep
  +
  1 half-down (holding weight in the half position for 5 seconds)
  1 half-down (hold for 4 seconds)
  1 half-down (hold for 3 seconds)
  1 half-down (hold for 2 seconds)
  1 half-down (hold for 1 second)
  +
  5 full reps

  15 seconds pause

(d) *Matrix Giant Steps Dumbbell Flyes*
   5 full reps
   +
   1 half-up
   2 half-down
   +
   3 full reps
   +
   4 half-up
   5 half-down
   +
   6 full reps

   15 seconds pause

(e) *Cumulative Matrix Alternates Dumbbell Flyes*

1 full rep		3 half-up
1 half-up		3 half-down
1 half-down		4 full reps
2 full reps	+	+
+		4 half-up
2 half-up		4 half-down
2 half-down		5 full reps
3 full reps		

   30 seconds pause

(f) *Conventional Dips*
   15 reps or as many as possible up to 15

   Finish

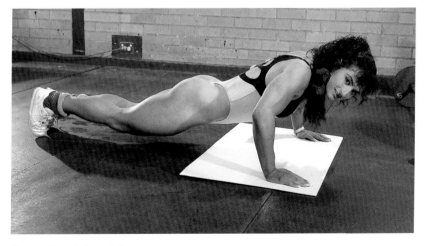

Conventional Floor Dip

Thigh Matrix

Stage 2

Sequence A

(a) *Matrix Giant Steps Squats*
    5 full reps
      +
    1 half-up
    2 half-down
      +
    3 full reps
      +
    4 half-up
    5 half-down
      +
    6 full reps

    40 seconds pause

(b) *Matrix Reversals Squats*
    5 full reps
      +
    1 rep 3/4 up
    1 rep 3/4 down
      +
    1 rep 3/4 up
    1 rep 3/4 down
      +
    1 rep 3/4 up
    1 rep 3/4 down
      +
    5 full reps

    50 seconds pause

(c) *Conventional Iso-Matrix Squats*
    5 full reps
      +
    5 half-up (hold for 5 seconds)
    5 half-down (hold for 5 seconds)
      +
    5 full reps

    60 seconds pause

(d) *Matrix Ladders Leg Press*

5 full reps		1 rep 1/5 down
+		1 rep 2/5 down
1 rep 1/5 up		1 rep 3/5 down
1 rep 2/5 up	+	1 rep 4/5 down
1 rep 3/5 up		1 full rep
1 rep 4/5 up		+
+		5 full reps
1 full rep		

30 seconds pause

(e) *Cumulative iso-Matrix Leg Press*
1 full rep
+
1 half-up (hold for 1 second)
2 half-up (hold each rep for 2 seconds)
3 half-up (hold each rep for 3 seconds)
4 half-up (hold each rep for 4 seconds)
+
5 full reps
+
1 half-down (hold for 1 second)
2 half-down (hold each rep for 2 seconds)
3 half-down (hold each rep for 3 seconds)
4 half-down (hold each rep for 4 seconds)
+
5 full reps

30 seconds pause

(f) *Cumulative Matrix Alternates Leg Press*

1 full rep		3 half-up
1 half-up		3 half-down
1 half-down		4 full reps
2 full reps	+	+
+		4 half-up
2 half-up		4 half-down
2 half-down		5 full reps
3 full reps		

35 seconds pause

(g) *Iso-Matrix Giant Steps Leg Press*
5 full reps
  +
1 half-up (hold for 5 seconds)
2 half-down (hold each rep for 4 seconds)
  +
3 full reps
  +
4 half-up (hold each rep for 3 seconds)
5 half-down (hold each rep for 2 seconds)
  +
6 full reps

3 minutes pause

Sequence B

(a) *Matrix Reversals Leg Curls*
5 full reps
  +
1 rep 3/4 up
1 rep 3/4 down
  +
1 rep 3/4 up
1 rep 3/4 down
  +
1 rep 3/4 up
1 rep 3/4 down
  +
5 full reps

15 seconds pause

(b) *Matrix Steps Leg Curls*
5 full reps
  +
1 half-up
2 half-down
3 half-up
4 half-down
5 half-up
6 half-down
  +
5 full reps

20 seconds pause

(c) *Cumulative Iso-Matrix Steps Leg Curls*
1 full rep
+
2 half-up (hold each rep for 3 seconds)
3 half-down (hold each rep for 4 seconds)
4 half-up (hold each rep for 5 seconds)
5 half-down (hold each rep for 6 seconds)
+
6 full reps

25 seconds pause

(d) *Cumulative Matrix Ladders Leg Curls*

1 full rep	1 rep 1/5 down
+	2 reps 2/5 down
1 rep 1/5 up	3 reps 3/5 down
2 reps 2/5 up	4 reps 4/5 down
3 reps 3/5 up +	+
4 reps 4/5 up	5 full reps
+	
5 full reps	

15 seconds pause

(e) *Matrix Giant Steps Squats*
5 full reps
+
1 half-up
2 half-down
+
3 full reps
+
4 half-up
5 half-down
+
6 full reps

15 seconds pause

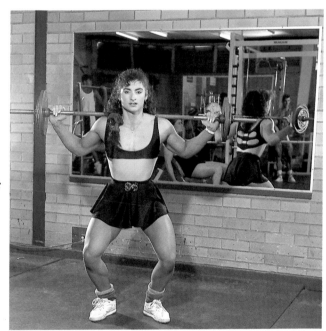

Matrix Giant Steps Squats

(f) *Ascending iso-Matrix Leg Extensions*
   5 full reps
   +
   1 half-up (holding weight in the half
   position for 1 second)
   1 half-up (hold for 2 seconds)
   1 half-up (hold for 3 seconds)
   1 half-up (hold for 4 seconds)
   1 half-up (hold for 5 seconds)
   1 full rep
   +
   1 half-down (holding weight in the
   half position for 1 second)
   1 half-down (hold for 2 seconds)
   1 half-down (hold for 3 seconds)
   1 half-down (hold for 4 seconds)
   1 half-down (hold for 5 seconds)
   +
   5 full reps

   20 seconds pause

(g) *Cumulative Matrix Alternates Leg Extensions*

1 full rep	3 half-up
1 half-up	3 half-down
1 half-down	4 full reps
2 full reps +	+
+	4 half-up
2 half-up	4 half-down
2 half-down	5 full reps
3 full reps	

   Finish

Biceps Matrix

Stage 2

Sequence A

(a) *Matrix Reversals Preacher Bench Curls*
    5 full reps
       +
    1 rep 3/4 up
    1 rep 3/4 down
       +
    1 rep 3/4 up
    1 rep 3/4 down
       +
    1 rep 3/4 up
    1 rep 3/4 down
       +
    5 full reps

    15 seconds pause

(b) *Matrix Steps Preacher Bench Curls*
    5 full reps
       +
    1 half-up
    2 half-down
    3 half-up
    4 half-down
    5 half-up
    6 half-down
       +
    5 full reps

    20 seconds pause

(c) *Matrix Alternates Preacher Bench Curls*

5 full reps		1 half-up
+		1 half-down
1 half-up		3 full reps
1 half-down		+
1 full rep	+	1 half-up
+		1 half-down
1 half-up		4 full reps
1 half-down		+
2 full reps		1 half-up
		1 half-down
		5 full reps

25 seconds pause

(d) *Iso-Matrix Steps Preacher Bench Curls*
   1 full rep
   +
   2 half-up (hold each rep for 3 seconds)
   3 half-down (hold each rep for 3 seconds)
   4 half-up (hold each rep for 3 seconds)
   5 half-down (hold each rep for 3 seconds)
   +
   6 full reps

   30 seconds pause

(e) *Iso-Matrix Giant Steps Incline Bench Dumbbell Curls*
   5 full reps
   +
   1 half-up (hold for 5 seconds)
   2 half-down (hold each rep for 4 seconds)
   +
   3 full reps
   +
   4 half-up (hold each rep for 3 seconds)
   5 half-down (hold each rep for 2 seconds)
   +
   6 full reps

   35 seconds pause

(f) *Matrix Ladders Incline Bench Dumbbell Curls*

5 full reps	1 rep 1/5 down
+	1 rep 2/5 down
1 rep 1/5 up	1 rep 3/5 down
1 rep 2/5 up +	1 rep 4/5 down
1 rep 3/5 up	1 full rep
1 rep 4/5 up	+
+	5 full reps
1 full rep	

40 seconds pause

(g) *Cumulative iso-Matrix Steps Incline Bench Dumbbell Curls*
1 full rep
+
2 half-up (hold each rep for 3 seconds)
3 half-down (hold each rep for 4 seconds)
4 half-up (hold each rep for 5 seconds)
5 half-down (hold each rep for 6 seconds)
+
6 full reps

3 minutes pause

Sequence B

(a) *Matrix Giant Steps Standing Barbell Curls*
5 full reps
+
1 half-up
2 half-down
+
3 full reps
+
4 half-up
5 half-down
+
6 full reps

15 seconds pause

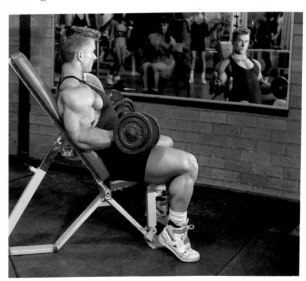

Cumulative iso-Matrix Steps Incline Bench Dumbbell Curls

(0) *Matrix Reversals Standing Barbell Curls*
   5 full reps
   +
   1 rep 3/4 up
   1 rep 3/4 down
   +
   1 rep 3/4 up
   1 rep 3/4 down
   +
   1 rep 3/4 up
   1 rep 3/4 down
   +
   5 full reps

   20 seconds pause

(c) *Iso-Matrix Steps Standing Barbell Curls*
   1 full rep
   +
   2 half-up (hold each rep for 3 seconds)
   3 half-down (hold each rep for 3 seconds)
   4 half-up (hold each rep for 3 seconds)
   5 half-down (hold each rep for 3 seconds)
   +
   6 full reps

   25 seconds pause

(d) *Matrix Alternates Standing Barbell Curls*

5 full reps		1 half-up
+		1 half-down
1 half-up		3 full reps
1 half-down		+
1 full rep	+	1 half-up
+		1 half-down
1 half-up		4 full reps
1 half-down		+
2 full reps		1 half-up
		1 half-down
		5 full reps

   Finish

Triceps Matrix

Stage 2

Sequence A

(a) *Matrix Giant Steps Triceps Pushdowns*
5 full reps
+
1 half-up
2 half-down
+
3 full reps
+
4 half-up
5 half-down
+
6 full reps

15 seconds pause

(b) *Matrix Alternates Triceps Pushdowns*

5 full reps		1 half-up
+		1 half-down
1 half-up		3 full reps
1 half-down		+
1 full rep	+	1 half-up
+		1 half-down
1 half-up		4 full reps
1 half-down		+
2 full reps		1 half-up
		1 half-down
		5 full reps

20 seconds pause

(c) *Matrix Reversals Triceps Pushdowns*
5 full reps
+
1 rep 3/4 up
1 rep 3/4 down
+
1 rep 3/4 up
1 rep 3/4 down
+
1 rep 3/4 up
1 rep 3/4 down
+
5 full reps

25 seconds pause

(d) *Conventional Matrix Dips*
5 full reps
5 half-up
5 half-down
5 full reps

30 seconds pause

(e) *Matrix Steps Dips*
5 full reps
+
1 half-up
2 half-down
3 half-up
4 half-down
5 half-up
6 half-down
+
5 full reps

40 seconds pause

(f) *Iso-Matrix Steps Triceps Pushdowns*
1 full rep
+
2 half-up (hold each rep for 3 seconds)
3 half-down (hold each rep for 3 seconds)
4 half-up (hold each rep for 3 seconds)
5 half-down (hold each rep for 3 seconds)
+
6 full reps

15 seconds pause

(g) *Matrix Ladders Triceps Pushdowns*

5 full reps	1 rep 1/5 down
+	1 rep 2/5 down
1 rep 1/5 up	1 rep 3/5 down
1 rep 2/5 up +	1 rep 4/5 down
1 rep 3/5 up	1 full rep
1 rep 4/5 up	+
+	5 full reps
1 full rep	

3 minutes pause

Sequence B

(a) *Matrix Steps Lying Triceps Press*
    5 full reps
    +
    1 half-up
    2 half-down
    3 half-up
    4 half-down
    5 half-up
    6 half-down
    +
    5 full reps

20 seconds pause

(b) *Cumulative Matrix Alternates Lying Triceps Press*

1 full rep	3 half-up
1 half-up	3 half-down
1 half-down	4 full reps
2 full reps +	+
+	4 half-up
2 half-up	4 half-down
2 half-down	5 full reps
3 full reps	

25 seconds pause

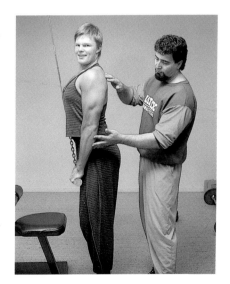

Leon Carlier practising Matrix
Ladders Triceps Pushdowns.

(c) *Matrix Reversals Lying Triceps Press*
5 full reps
+
1 rep 3/4 up
1 rep 3/4 down
+
1 rep 3/4 up
1 rep 3/4 down
+
1 rep 3/4 up
1 rep 3/4 down
+
5 full reps

25 seconds pause

(d) *Matrix Alternates Standing Overhead Triceps Press*

5 full reps		1 half-up
+		1 half-down
1 half-up		3 full reps
1 half-down		+
1 full rep	+	1 half-up
+		1 half-down
1 half-up		4 full reps
1 half-down		+
2 full reps		1 half-up
		1 half-down
		5 full reps

25 seconds pause

(e) *Cumulative Matrix Ladders Lying Triceps Press*

1 full rep		1 rep 1/5 down
+		2 reps 2/5 down
1 rep 1/5 up		3 reps 3/5 down
2 reps 2/5 up		4 reps 4/5 down
3 reps 3/5 up	+	+
4 reps 4/5 up		5 full reps
+		
5 full reps		

Finish

Deltoid Matrix

Stage 2

Sequence A

(a) *Matrix Dumbbell Roll Press*
   15 reps

   20 seconds pause

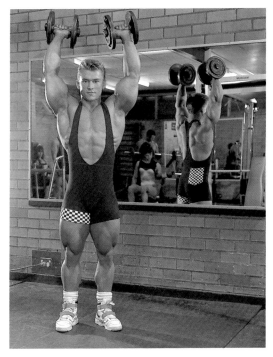

Matrix Dumbbell Roll Press

(b) *Iso-Matrix Giant Steps Press Behind the Neck*
   5 full reps
      +
   1 half-up (hold for 5 seconds)
   2 half-down (hold each rep for 4 seconds)
      +
   3 full reps
      +
   4 half-up (hold each rep for 3 seconds)
   5 half-down (hold each rep for 2 seconds)
      +
   6 full reps

   25 seconds pause

(c) *Matrix Reversals Press In Front of the Neck*
    5 full reps
        +
    1 rep 3/4 up
    1 rep 3/4 down
        +
    1 rep 3/4 up
    1 rep 3/4 down
        +
    1 rep 3/4 up
    1 rep 3/4 down
        +
    5 full reps

    30 seconds pause

(d) *Matrix Giant Steps Press Behind the Neck*
    5 full reps
        +
    1 half-up
    2 half-down
        +
    3 full reps
        +
    4 half-up
    5 half-down
        +
    6 full reps

    20 seconds pause

(e) *Matrix Steps Upright Rows*
    5 full reps
        +
    1 half-up
    2 half-down
    3 half-up
    4 half-down
    5 half-up
    6 half-down
        +
    5 full reps

    15 seconds pause

(f) *Matrix Ladders Upright Rows*

5 full reps		1 rep 1/5 down
+		1 rep 2/5 down
1 rep 1/5 up		1 rep 3/5 down
1 rep 2/5 up	+	1 rep 4/5 down
1 rep 3/5 up		1 full rep
1 rep 4/5 up		+
+		5 full reps
1 full rep		

20 seconds pause

(g) *Cumulative iso-Matrix Steps Upright Rows*
1 full rep
+
2 half-up (hold each rep for 3 seconds)
3 half-down (hold each rep for 4 seconds)
4 half-up (hold each rep for 5 seconds)
5 half-down (hold each rep for 6 seconds)
+
6 full reps

25 seconds pause

(h) *Matrix Alternates Upright Rows*

5 full reps		1 half-up
+		1 half-down
1 half-up		3 full reps
1 half-down	+	+
1 full rep		1 half-up
+		1 half-down
1 half-up		4 full reps
1 half-down		+
2 full reps		1 half-up
		1 half-down
		5 full reps

2 minutes pause

Sequence B

(a) *Matrix Roll Presses*
15 full reps

20 seconds pause

(b) *Cumulative iso-Matrix Steps Dumbbell Lateral Raises*
    1 full rep
        +
    2 half-up (hold each rep for 3 seconds)
    3 half-down (hold each rep for 4 seconds)
    4 half-up (hold each rep for 5 seconds)
    5 half-down (hold each rep for 6 seconds)
        +
    6 full reps

    15 seconds pause

(c) *Matrix Giant Steps Dumbbell Front Raises*
    5 full reps
        +
    1 half-up
    2 half-down
        +
    3 full reps
        +
    4 half-up
    5 half-down
        +
    6 full reps

    20 seconds pause

(d) *Matrix Reversals Dumbbell Lateral Raises*
    5 full reps
        +
    1 rep 3/4 up
    1 rep 3/4 down
        +
    1 rep 3/4 up
    1 rep 3/4 down
        +
    1 rep 3/4 up
    1 rep 3/4 down
        +
    5 full reps

    25 seconds pause

(e) *Iso-Matrix Giant Steps Dumbbell Front Raises*
    5 full reps
       +
    1 half-up (hold for 5 seconds)
    2 half-down (hold each rep for 4 seconds)
       +
    3 full reps
       +
    4 half-up (hold each rep for 3 seconds)
    5 half-down (hold each rep for 2 seconds)
       +
    6 full reps

    30 seconds pause

(f) *Matrix Roll Presses*
    15 full reps

    Finish

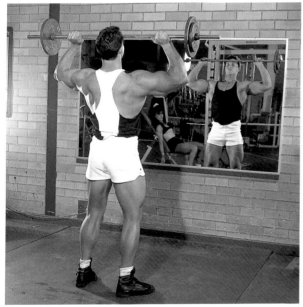

Matrix Roll Presses

Lats and Back Matrix

Stage 2

Sequence A

(a) *Matrix Alternates Lat Machine Pulldowns*

5 full reps	1 half-up
+	1 half-down
1 half-up	3 full reps
1 half-down +	+
1 full rep	1 half-up
+	1 half-down
1 half-up	4 full reps
1 half-down	+
2 full reps	1 half-up
	1 half-down
	5 full reps

20 seconds pause

(b) *Cumulative iso-Matrix Steps Lat Machine Pulldowns*
   1 full rep
   +
   2 half-up (hold each rep for 3 seconds)
   3 half-down (hold each rep for 4 seconds)
   4 half-up (hold each rep for 5 seconds)
   5 half-down (hold each rep for 6 seconds)
   +
   6 full reps

25 seconds pause

(c) *Matrix Reversals Chin-Ups in Front of the Neck*
   5 full reps
   +
   1 rep 3/4 up
   1 rep 3/4 down
   +
   1 rep 3/4 up
   1 rep 3/4 down
   +
   1 rep 3/4 up
   1 rep 3/4 down
   +
   5 full reps

20 seconds pause

(d) *Matrix Steps Lat Machine Pulldowns*
　　5 full reps
　　　+
　　1 half-up
　　2 half-down
　　3 half-up
　　4 half-down
　　5 half-up
　　6 half-down
　　　+
　　5 full reps

　　30 seconds pause

(e) *Matrix Reversals Chin-Ups Behind the Neck*
　　3 full reps
　　　+
　　1 rep 3/4 up
　　1 rep 3/4 down
　　　+
　　1 rep 3/4 up
　　1 rep 3/4 down
　　　+
　　1 rep 3/4 up
　　1 rep 3/4 down
　　　+
　　3 full reps

　　20 seconds pause

(f) *Bent-Arm Pullovers*
　　12 reps or as many as possible up to 12

　　20 seconds pause

(g) *Matrix Giant Steps Lat Machine Pulldowns*
　　5 full reps
　　　+
　　1 half-up
　　2 half-down
　　　+
　　3 full reps
　　　+
　　4 half-up
　　5 half-down
　　　+
　　6 full reps

　　3 minutes pause

Sequence B

(a) *Bent-Arm Pullovers*
     12 reps or as many as possible up to 12

     20 seconds pause

(b) *Matrix Giant Steps Bent-Over Rows*
     5 full reps
       +
     1 half-up
     2 half-down
       +
     3 full reps
       +
     4 half-up
     5 half-down
       +
     6 full reps

     25 seconds pause

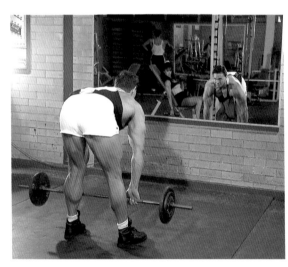

Iso-Matrix Steps Bent-Over Rows

(c) *Iso-Matrix Steps Bent-Over Rows*
     1 full rep
       +
     2 half-up (hold each rep for 3 seconds)
     3 half-down (hold each rep for 3 seconds)
     4 half-up (hold each rep for 3 seconds)
     5 half-down (hold each rep for 3 seconds)
       +
     6 full reps

     30 seconds pause

(d) *Conventional Bent-Arm Pullovers*
12 reps or as many as possible up to 12

20 seconds pause

(e) *Ascending iso-Matrix Bent-Over Rows*
5 full reps
+
1 half-up (holding weight in the half position for 1 second)
1 half-up (hold for 2 seconds)
1 half-up (hold for 3 seconds)
1 half-up (hold for 4 seconds)
1 half-up (hold for 5 seconds)
1 full rep
+
1 half-down (holding weight in the half position for 1 second)
1 half-down (hold for 2 seconds)
1 half-down (hold for 3 seconds)
1 half-down (hold for 4 seconds)
1 half-down (hold for 5 seconds)
+
5 full reps

25 seconds pause

(f) *Matrix Steps Bent-Over Rows*
5 full reps
+
1 half-up
2 half-down
3 half-up
4 half-down
5 half-up
6 half-down
+
5 full reps

Finish

III Matrix core routines: weeks 25–36

Chest Matrix

Stage 3

Sequence A

(a) *Descending Matrix Reversals Bench Press*
7 full reps
+
1 rep 3/4 up
1 rep 3/4 down
+
6 full reps
+
1 rep 3/4 up
1 rep 3/4 down
+
5 full reps

20 seconds pause

(b) *Iso-Matrix Giant Steps Bench Press*
5 full reps
+
1 half-up (hold for 5 seconds)
2 half-down (hold each rep for 4 seconds)
+
3 full reps
+
4 half-up (hold each rep for 3 seconds)
5 half-down (hold each rep for 2 seconds)
+
6 full reps

25 seconds pause

(c) *Matrix Reversals Bench Press*
5 full reps
+
1 rep 3/4 up
1 rep 3/4 down
+
1 rep 3/4 up
1 rep 3/4 down
+
1 rep 3/4 up
1 rep 3/4 down
+
5 full reps

30 seconds pause

(d) *Matrix Giant Steps Bench Press*
5 full reps
+
1 half-up
2 half-down
+
3 full reps
+
4 half-up
5 half-down
+
6 full reps

35 seconds pause

(e) *Ascending Matrix Reversals Incline Press*
5 full reps
+
1 rep 3/4 up
1 rep 3/4 down
+
6 full reps
+
1 rep 3/4 up
1 rep 3/4 down
+
7 full reps

30 seconds pause

(f) *Cumulative Matrix Ladders Incline Press*

1 full rep	1 rep 1/5 down
+	2 reps 2/5 down
1 rep 1/5 up	3 reps 3/5 down
2 reps 2/5 up	4 reps 4/5 down
3 reps 3/5 up +	+
4 reps 4/5 up	5 full reps
+	
5 full reps	

25 seconds pause

(g) *Cumulative iso-Matrix Steps Incline Press*
1 full rep
+
2 half-up (hold each rep for 3 seconds)
3 half-down (hold each rep for 4 seconds)
4 half-up (hold each rep for 5 seconds)
5 half-down (hold each rep for 6 seconds)
+
6 full reps

3 minutes pause

Sequence B

(a) *Matrix Steps Dips*
5 full reps
+
1 half-up
2 half-down
3 half-up
4 half-down
5 half-up
6 half-down
+
5 full reps

15 seconds pause

(b) *Conventional Matrix Floor Push-Ups*
5 full reps
5 half-up
5 half-down
5 full reps

20 seconds pause

(c) *Cumulative Matrix Reversals Incline Bench Press*
  3 full reps
    +
  3 reps 3/4 up
  3 reps 3/4 down
    +
  4 full reps
    +
  4 reps 3/4 up
  4 reps 3/4 down
    +
  5 full reps

  25 seconds pause

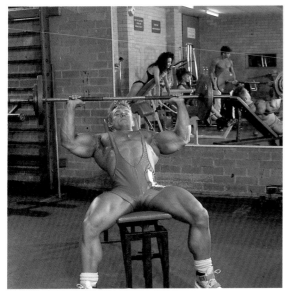

Cumulative Matrix Reversals
Incline Bench Press

(d) *Iso-Matrix Giant Steps Pec Deck*
  5 full reps
    +
  1 half-up (hold for 5 seconds)
  2 half-down (hold each rep for 4 seconds)
    +
  3 full reps
    +
  4 half-up (hold each rep for 3 seconds)
  5 half-down (hold each rep for 2 seconds)
    +
  6 full reps

  30 seconds pause

(e) *Matrix Giant Steps Pec Deck*
5 full reps
+
1 half-up
2 half-down
+
3 full reps
+
4 half-up
5 half-down
+
6 full reps

35 seconds pause

(f) *Matrix Reversals Pec Deck*
5 full reps
+
1 rep 3/4 up
1 rep 3/4 down
+
1 rep 3/4 up
1 rep 3/4 down
+
1 rep 3/4 up
1 rep 3/4 down
+
5 full reps

Finish

Thigh Matrix

Stage 3

Sequence A

(a) *Matrix Reversals Leg Press*
5 full reps
+
1 rep 3/4 up
1 rep 3/4 down
+
1 rep 3/4 up
1 rep 3/4 down
+
1 rep 3/4 up
1 rep 3/4 down
+
5 full reps

15 seconds pause

(b) *Iso-Matrix Steps Leg Press*
1 full rep
+
2 half-up (hold each rep for 3 seconds)
3 half-down (hold each rep for 3 seconds)
4 half-up (hold each rep for 3 seconds)
5 half-down (hold each rep for 3 seconds)
+
6 full reps

20 seconds pause

(c) *Descending Matrix Reversals Leg Press*
7 full reps
+
1 rep 3/4 up
1 rep 3/4 down
+
6 full reps
+
1 rep 3/4 up
1 rep 3/4 down
+
5 full reps

25 seconds pause

(d) *Cumulative iso-Matrix Steps Leg Press*
   1 full rep
      +
   2 half-up (hold each rep for 3 seconds)
   3 half-down (hold each rep for 4 seconds)
   4 half up (hold each rep for 5 seconds)
   5 half-down (hold each rep for 6 seconds)
      +
   6 full reps

   30 seconds pause

(e) *Matrix Steps Squats*
   5 full reps
      +
   1 half-up
   2 half-down
   3 half-up
   4 half-down
   5 half-up
   6 half-down
      +
   5 full reps

   20 seconds pause

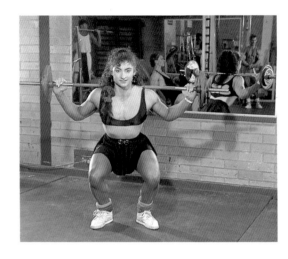

Matrix Steps Squats

(f) *Matrix Alternates Leg Extensions*

5 full reps	1 half-up
+	1 half-down
1 half-up	3 full reps
1 half-down	+
1 full rep +	1 half-up
+	1 half-down
1 half-up	4 full reps
1 half-down	+
2 full reps	1 half-up
	1 half-down
	5 full reps

   25 seconds pause

(g) *Cumulative Matrix Reversals Leg Extensions*
3 full reps
+
3 reps 3/4 up
3 reps 3/4 down
+
4 full reps
+
4 reps 3/4 up
4 reps 3/4 down
+
5 full reps

3 minutes pause

Sequence B

(a) *Matrix Giant Steps Squat*
5 full reps
+
1 half-up
2 half-down
+
3 full reps
+
4 half-up
5 half-down
+
6 full reps

25 seconds pause

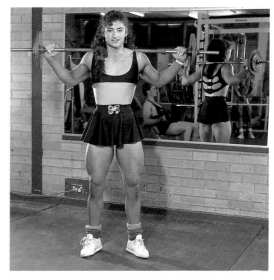

Cumulative Matrix Reversals Leg Extensions

(b) *Matrix Reversals Squat*
5 full reps
+
1 rep 3/4 up
1 rep 3/4 down
+
1 rep 3/4 up
1 rep 3/4 down
+
1 rep 3/4 up
1 rep 3/4 down
+
5 full reps

25 seconds pause

(c) *Cumulative iso-Matrix Steps Leg Curls*
1 full rep
+
2 half-up (hold each rep for 3 seconds)
3 half-down (hold each rep for 4 seconds)
4 half-up (hold each rep for 5 seconds)
5 half-down (hold each rep for 6 seconds)
+
6 full reps

30 seconds pause

(d) *Ascending Matrix Reversals Leg Curls*
5 full reps
+
1 rep 3/4 up
1 rep 3/4 down
+
6 full reps
+
1 rep 3/4 up
1 rep 3/4 down
+
7 full reps

30 seconds pause

(e) *Matrix Alternates Squat*

5 full reps		1 half-up
+		1 half-down
1 half-up		3 full reps
1 half-down		+
1 full rep	+	1 half-up
+		1 half-down
1 half-up		4 full reps
1 half-down		+
2 full reps		1 half-up
		1 half-down
		5 full reps

50 seconds pause

(f) *Cumulative Matrix Ladders Squat*

1 full rep	1 rep 1/5 down
+	2 reps 2/5 down
1 rep 1/5 up	3 reps 3/5 down
2 reps 2/5 up	4 reps 4/5 down
3 reps 3/5 up +	+
4 reps 4/5 up	5 full reps
+	
5 full reps	

Finish

Biceps Matrix

Stage 3

Sequence A

(a) *Matrix Reversals Standing Barbell Curls*

5 full reps

+

1 rep 3/4 up
1 rep 3/4 down

+

1 rep 3/4 up
1 rep 3/4 down

+

1 rep 3/4 up
1 rep 3/4 down

+

5 full reps

20 seconds pause

(b) *Iso-Matrix Giant Steps Standing Barbell Curls*

5 full reps

+

1 half-up (hold for 5 seconds)
2 half-down (hold each rep for 4 seconds)

+

3 full reps

+

4 half-up (hold each rep for 3 seconds)
5 half-down (hold each rep for 2 seconds)

+

6 full reps

25 seconds pause

(c) *Matrix Giant Steps Incline Bench Dumbbell Curls*
    5 full reps
    +
    1 half-up
    2 half-down
    +
    3 full reps
    +
    4 half-up
    5 half-down
    +
    6 full reps

    30 seconds pause

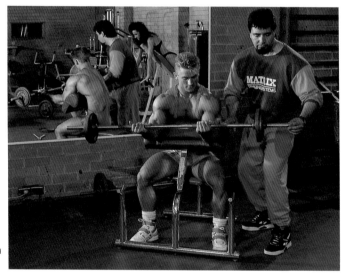

Matrix Preacher Bench
Curls

(d) *Cumulative Matrix Alternates Incline Bench Dumbbell Curls*

1 full rep	3 half-up
1 half-up	3 half-down
1 half-down	4 full reps
2 full reps +	+
+	4 half-up
2 half-up	4 half-down
2 half-down	5 full reps
3 full reps	

    30 seconds pause

(e) *Cumulative iso-Matrix Steps Preacher Bench Curls*
    1 full rep
      +
    2 half-up (hold each rep for 3 seconds)
    3 half-down (hold each rep for 4 seconds)
    4 half-up (hold each rep for 5 seconds)
    5 half-down (hold each rep for 6 seconds)
      +
    6 full reps

    35 seconds pause

(f) *Descending Matrix Reversals Preacher Bench Curls*
    7 full reps
      +
    1 rep 3/4 up
    1 rep 3/4 down
      +
    6 full reps
      +
    1 rep 3/4 up
    1 rep 3/4 down
      +
    5 full reps

    3 minutes pause

Sequence B

(a) *Cumulative Matrix Reversals Incline Bench Dumbbell Curls*
    3 full reps
      +
    3 reps 3/4 up
    3 reps 3/4 down
      +
    4 full reps
      +
    4 reps 3/4 up
    4 reps 3/4 down
      +
    5 full reps

    20 seconds pause

(b) *Iso-Matrix Steps Incline Bench Dumbbell Curls*
1 full rep
+
2 half-up (hold each rep for 3 seconds)
3 half-down (hold each rep for 3 seconds)
4 half-up (hold each rep for 3 seconds)
5 half-down (hold each rep for 3 seconds)
+
6 full reps

25 seconds pause

(c) *Descending Matrix Reversals Standing Barbell Curls*
7 full reps
+
1 rep 3/4 up
1 rep 3/4 down
+
6 full reps
+
1 rep 3/4 up
1 rep 3/4 down
+
5 full reps

30 seconds pause

(d) *Iso-Matrix Giant Steps Standing Barbell Curls*
5 full reps
+
1 half-up (hold for 5 seconds)
2 half-down (hold each rep for 4 seconds)
+
3 full reps
+
4 half-up (hold each rep for 3 seconds)
5 half-down (hold each rep for 2 seconds)
+
6 full reps

30 seconds pause

(e) *Matrix Giant Steps Preacher Bench Curls*
5 full reps
+
1 half-up
2 half-down
+
3 full reps
+
4 half-up
5 half-down
+
6 full reps

35 seconds pause

(f) *Ascending Matrix Reversals Preacher Bench Curls*
5 full reps
+
1 rep 3/4 up
1 rep 3/4 down
+
6 full reps
+
1 rep 3/4 up
1 rep 3/4 down
+
7 full reps

Finish

Triceps Matrix

Stage 3

Sequence A

(a) *Cumulative Matrix Reversals Lying Triceps Press*
3 full reps
+
3 reps 3/4 up
3 reps 3/4 down
+
4 full reps
+
4 reps 3/4 up
4 reps 3/4 down
+
5 full reps

20 seconds pause

(b) *Matrix Giant Steps Lying Triceps Press*
5 full reps
+
1 half-up
2 half-down
+
3 full reps
+
4 half-up
5 half-down
+
6 full reps

20 seconds pause

(c) *Iso-Matrix Steps Lying Triceps Press*
1 full rep
+
2 half-up (hold each rep for 3 seconds)
3 half-down (hold each rep for 3 seconds)
4 half-up (hold each rep for 3 seconds)
5 half-down (hold each rep for 3 seconds)
+
6 full reps

30 seconds pause

(d) *Matrix Steps Lying Triceps Press*
5 full reps
    +
1 half-up
2 half-down
3 half-up
4 half-down
5 half-up
6 half-down
    +
5 full reps

30 seconds pause

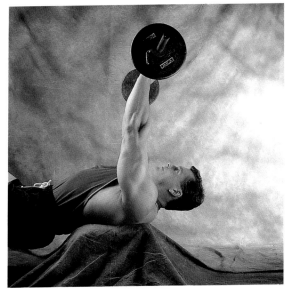

Matrix Lying Triceps Press

(e) *Descending Matrix Reversals Triceps Pushdowns*
7 full reps
    +
1 rep 3/4 up
1 rep 3/4 down
    +
6 full reps
    +
1 rep 3/4 up
1 rep 3/4 down
    +
5 full reps

25 seconds pause

(f) *Cumulative iso-Matrix Triceps Pushdowns*
1 full rep
+
1 half-up (hold for 1 second)
2 half-up (hold each rep for 2 seconds)
3 half-up (hold each rep for 3 seconds)
4 half-up (hold each rep for 4 seconds)
+
5 full reps
+
1 half-down (hold for 1 second)
2 half-down (hold each rep for 2 seconds)
3 half-down (hold each rep for 3 seconds)
4 half-down (hold each rep for 4 seconds)
+
5 full reps

25 seconds pause

(g) *Matrix Alternates Triceps Pushdowns*

5 full reps		1 half-up
+		1 half-down
1 half-up		3 full reps
1 half-down		+
1 full rep	+	1 half-up
+		1 half-down
1 half-up		4 full reps
1 half-down		+
2 full reps		1 half-up
		1 half-down
		5 full reps

3 minutes pause

Sequence B

(a) *Matrix Reversals Standing Overhead Triceps Press*
5 full reps
+
1 rep 3/4 up
1 rep 3/4 down
+
1 rep 3/4 up
1 rep 3/4 down
+
1 rep 3/4 up
1 rep 3/4 down
+
5 full reps

20 seconds pause

(b) *Dips*
15 reps or as many as possible up to 15

20 seconds pause

(c) *Matrix Giant Steps Standing Overhead Triceps Press*
5 full reps
+
1 half-up
2 half-down
+
3 full reps
+
4 half-up
5 half-down
+
6 full reps

25 seconds pause

(d) *Dips*
15 reps or as many as possible up to 15

30 seconds pause

(e) *Ascending Matrix Reversals Standing Triceps Press*
5 full reps
+
1 rep 3/4 up
1 rep 3/4 down
+
6 full reps
+
1 rep 3/4 up
1 rep 3/4 down
+
7 full reps

30 seconds pause

(f) *Dips*
15 reps or as many as possible up to 15

Finish

Deltoid Matrix

Stage 3

Sequence A

(a) *Matrix Roll Press*
15 full reps

20 seconds pause

(b) *Matrix Reversals Dumbbell Lateral Raises*
5 full reps
+
1 rep 3/4 up
1 rep 3/4 down
+
1 rep 3/4 up
1 rep 3/4 down
+
1 rep 3/4 up
1 rep 3/4 down
+
5 full reps

20 seconds pause

Tony Webber performing a
Matrix Roll Press.

(c) *Matrix Giant Steps Dumbbell Lateral Raises*
   5 full reps
   +
   1 half-up
   2 half-down
   +
   3 full reps
   +
   4 half-up
   5 half-down
   +
   6 full reps

   20 seconds pause

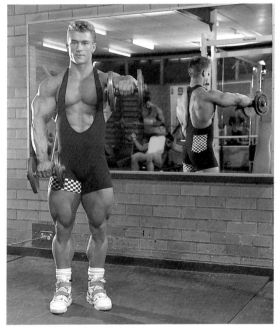

Iso-Matrix Steps Dumbbell Front
Raises

(d) *Iso-Matrix Steps Dumbbell Front Raises*
   1 full rep
   +
   2 half-up (hold each rep for 3 seconds)
   3 half-down (hold each rep for 3 seconds)
   4 half-up (hold each rep for 3 seconds)
   5 half-down (hold each rep for 3 seconds)
   +
   6 full reps

   30 seconds pause

(e) *Descending Matrix Reversals Dumbbell Front Raises*
7 full reps
+
1 rep 3/4 up
1 rep 3/4 down
+
6 full reps
+
1 rep 3/4 up
1 rep 3/4 down
+
5 full reps

30 seconds pause

(f) *Matrix Steps Press Behind the Neck*
5 full reps
+
1 half-up
2 half-down
3 half-up
4 half-down
5 half-up
6 half-down
+
5 full reps

35 seconds pause

(g) *Cumulative iso-Matrix Steps Press in Front of the Neck*
1 full rep
+
2 half-up (hold each rep for 3 seconds)
3 half-down (hold each rep for 4 seconds)
4 half-up (hold each rep for 5 seconds)
5 half-down (hold each rep for 6 seconds)
+
6 full reps

40 seconds pause

(h) *Cumulative Matrix Reversals Press Behind the Neck*
3 full reps
+
3 reps 3/4 up
3 reps 3/4 down
+
4 full reps
+
4 reps 3/4 up
4 reps 3/4 down
+
5 full reps

50 seconds pause

(i) *Matrix Giant Steps Press in Front of the Neck*
5 full reps
+
1 half-up
2 half-down
+
3 full reps
+
4 half-up
5 half-down
+
6 full reps

3 minutes pause

Sequence B

(a) *Matrix Roll Presses*
15 full reps

20 seconds pause

(b) *Matrix Giant Steps Upright Rows*
   5 full reps
      +
   1 half-up
   2 half-down
      +
   3 full reps
      +
   4 half-up
   5 half-down
      +
   6 full reps

   20 seconds pause

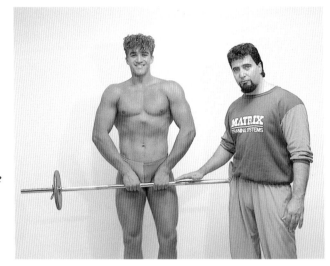

Matrix Upright Rows

(c) *Cumulative iso-Matrix Steps Upright Rows*
   1 full rep
      +
   2 half-up (hold each rep for 3 seconds)
   3 half-down (hold each rep for 4 seconds)
   4 half-up (hold each rep for 5 seconds)
   5 half-down (hold each rep for 6 seconds)
      +
   6 full reps

   30 seconds pause

(d) *Matrix Reversals Upright Rows*
   5 full reps
      +
   1 rep 3/4 up
   1 rep 3/4 down
      +
   1 rep 3/4 up
   1 rep 3/4 down
      +
   1 rep 3/4 up
   1 rep 3/4 down
      +
   5 full reps

   30 seconds pause

(e) *Iso-Matrix Giant Steps Upright Rows*
     5 full reps
        +
     1 half-up (hold for 5 seconds)
     2 half-down (hold each rep for 4 seconds)
        +
     3 full reps
        +
     4 half-up (hold each rep for 3 seconds)
     5 half-down (hold each rep for 2 seconds)
        +
     6 full reps

     20 seconds pause

(f) *Matrix Roll Press*
     15 full reps or as many as possible up to 15

     Finish

Lats and Back Matrix

Stage 3

Sequence A

(a) *Matrix Reversals Lat Machine Pulldowns*
   5 full reps
      +
   1 rep 3/4 up
   1 rep 3/4 down
      +
   1 rep 3/4 up
   1 rep 3/4 down
      +
   1 rep 3/4 up
   1 rep 3/4 down
      +
   5 full reps

   15 seconds pause

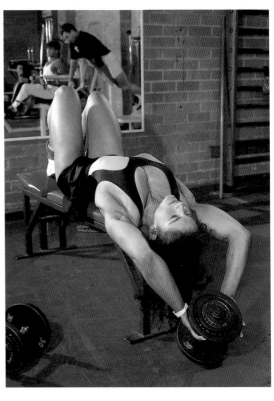

Bent-Arm Pullovers

(b) *Iso-Matrix Giant Steps Lat Machine Pulldowns in Front of the Neck*
   5 full reps
      +
   1 half-up (hold for 5 seconds)
   2 half-down (hold each rep for 4 seconds)
      +
   3 full reps
      +
   4 half-up (hold each rep for 3 seconds)
   5 half-down (hold each rep for 2 seconds)
      +
   6 full reps

   20 seconds pause

(c) *Matrix Giant Steps Lat Machine Pulldowns*
5 full reps
+
1 half-up
2 half-down
+
3 full reps
+
4 half-up
5 half-down
+
6 full reps

20 seconds pause

(d) *Cumulative Matrix Alternates Lat Machine Pulldowns in Front of the Neck*

1 full rep   3 half-up
1 half-up   3 half-down
1 half-down   4 full reps
2 full reps   +   +
+   4 half-up
2 half-up   4 half-down
2 half-down   5 full reps
2 full reps

25 seconds pause

(e) *Iso-Matrix Steps Bent-Over Rows*
1 full rep
+
2 half-up (hold each rep for 3 seconds)
3 half-down (hold each rep for 3 seconds)
4 half-up (hold each rep for 3 seconds)
5 half-down (hold each rep for 3 seconds)
+
6 full reps

30 seconds pause

(f) *Bent-Arm Pullovers*
12 reps or as many as possible up to 12

30 seconds pause

(g) *Cumulative Matrix Ladders Bent-Over Rows*

1 full rep	1 rep 1/5 down
+	2 reps 2/5 down
1 rep 1/5 up	3 reps 3/5 down
2 reps 2/5 up	4 reps 4/5 down
3 reps 3/5 up +	+
4 reps 4/5 up	5 full reps
+	
5 full reps	

35 seconds pause

(h) **Bent-Arm Pullovers**
12 reps or as many as possible up to 12

40 seconds pause

(i) *Matrix Alternates Bent-Over Rows*

5 full reps	1 half-up
+	1 half-down
1 half-up	3 full reps
1 half-down	+
1 full rep +	1 half-up
+	1 half-down
1 half-up	4 full reps
1 half-down	+
2 full reps	1 half-up
	1 half-doen
	5 full reps

3 minutes pause

Sequence B

(a) *Chin-Ups In Front of the Neck*
12 reps or as many as possible up to 12

20 seconds pause

(b) *Matrix Reversals Hyperextensions*
    5 full reps
       +
    1 rep 3/4 up
    1 rep 3/4 down
       +
    1 rep 3/4 up
    1 rep 3/4 down
       +
    1 rep 3/4 up
    1 rep 3/4 down
       +
    5 full reps

    20 seconds pause

(c) *Iso-Matrix Giant Steps Hyperextensions*
    5 full reps
       +
    1 half-up (hold for 5 seconds)
    2 half-down (hold each rep for 4 seconds)
       +
    3 full reps
       +
    4 half-up (hold each rep for 3 seconds)
    5 half-down (hold each rep for 2 seconds)
       +
    6 full reps

    20 seconds pause

(d) *Chin-Ups in Front of the Neck*
    12 reps or as many as possible up to 12

    20 seconds pause

(e) *Stiff-Legged Deadlifts*
    15 reps

    20 seconds pause

(f) *Chin-Ups Behind the Neck*
    12 reps or as many as possible up to 12

    20 seconds pause

(g) *Cumulative Matrix Reversals Bent-Over Rows*
   3 full reps
      +
   3 reps 3/4 up
   3 reps 3/4 down
      +
   4 full reps
      +
   4 reps 3/4 up
   4 reps 3/4 down
      +
   5 full reps

   25 seconds pause

(h) *Matrix Steps Bent-Over Rows*
   5 full reps
      +
   1 half-up (hold for 5 seconds)
   2 half-down (hold each rep for 4 seconds)
      +
   3 full reps
      +
   4 half-up (hold each rep for 3 seconds)
   5 half-down (hold each rep for 2 seconds)
      +
   6 full reps

   Finish

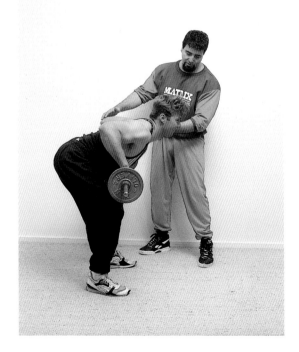

Cumulative Matrix Reversals
Bent-Over Rows

IV Matrix core routines: weeks 37–48

Chest Matrix

Stage 4

Sequence A

(a) *Matrix Composites Dumbbell Flyes*
    5 full reps
    +
    3 half-up
    3 half-down
    +
    3 half-up
    3 half-down
    +
    3 half-up
    3 half-down
    +
    5 full reps

    20 seconds pause

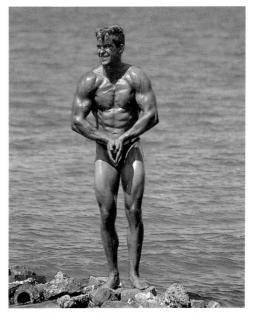

Jamie Palmer exhibits his remarkable chest development.

(b) *Matrix Composites Decline Bench Press*
    5 full reps
    +
    3 half-up
    3 half-down
    +
    3 half-up
    3 half-down
    +
    3 half-up
    3 half-down
    +
    5 full reps

    25 seconds pause

(c) *Matrix Reverse Ladders Bench Press*
5 full reps
+
1 rep 1/5 up
1 rep 1/5 down
+
1 rep 2/5 up
1 rep 2/5 down
+
1 rep 3/5 up
1 rep 3/5 down
+
1 rep 4/5 up
1 rep 4/5 down
+
5 full reps
25 seconds pause

(d) *Iso-Matrix Steps Incline Press*
1 full rep
+
2 half-up (hold each rep for 3 seconds)
3 half-down (hold each rep for 3 seconds)
4 half-up (hold each rep for 3 seconds)
5 half-down (hold each rep for 3 seconds)
+
6 full reps
25 seconds pause

(e) *Matrix Reverse Step Ladders Bench Press*
1 full rep
+
2 reps 1/5 up
3 reps 1/5 down
+
4 reps 2/5 up
5 reps 2/5 down
+
6 reps 3/5 up
7 reps 3/5 down
+
8 reps 4/5 up
9 reps 4/5 down
+
10 full reps
30 seconds pause

(f) *Iso-Matrix Giant Steps Bench Press*
5 full reps
+
1 half-up (hold for 5 seconds)
2 half-down (hold each rep for 4 seconds)
+
3 full reps
+
4 half-up (hold each rep for 3 seconds)
5 half-down (hold each rep for 2 seconds)
+
6 full reps

30 seconds pause

(g) *Matrix Composites Incline Press*
5 full reps
+
3 half-up
3 half-down
+
3 half-up
3 half-down
+
3 half-up
3 half-down
+
5 full reps

35 seconds pause

(h) *Cumulative iso-Matrix Steps Dumbbell Flyes*
1 full rep
+
2 half-up (hold each rep for 3 seconds)
3 half-down (hold each rep for 4 seconds)
4 half-up (hold each rep for 5 seconds)
5 half-down (hold each rep for 6 seconds)
+
6 full reps

35 seconds pause

(i) *Conventional Dips*
12 reps or as many as possible up to 12

3 minutes pause

Sequence B

(a) *Matrix Reverse Ladders Pec Deck*
   5 full reps
   +
   1 rep 1/5 up
   1 rep 1/5 down
   +
   1 rep 2/5 up
   1 rep 2/5 down
   +
   1 rep 3/5 up
   1 rep 3/5 down
   +
   1 rep 4/5 up
   1 rep 4/5 down
   +
   5 full reps

   20 seconds pause

(b) *Matrix Composites Pec Deck*
   5 full reps
   +
   3 half-up
   3 half-down
   +
   3 half-up
   3 half-down
   +
   3 half-up
   3 half-down
   +
   5 full reps

   20 seconds pause

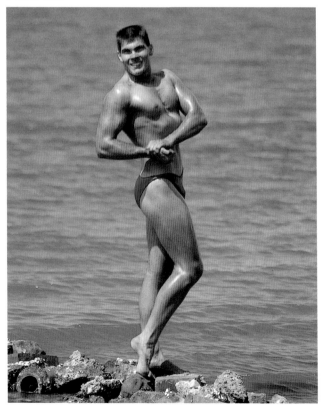

Seventeen-year-old Peter
Butler shows off his
Matrix-built chest.

(c) *Matrix Reverse Step Ladders Bench Press*
1 full rep
+
2 reps 1/5 up
3 reps 1/5 down
+
4 reps 2/5 up
5 reps 2/5 down
+
6 reps 3/5 up
7 reps 3/5 down
+
8 reps 4/5 up
9 reps 4/5 down
+
1 full rep

25 seconds pause

(d) *Iso-Matrix Giant Steps Bench Press*
5 full reps
+
1 half-up (hold for 5 seconds)
2 half-down (hold each rep for 4 seconds)
+
3 full reps
+
4 half-up (hold each rep for 3 seconds)
5 half-down (hold each rep for 2 seconds)
+
6 full reps

25 seconds pause

(e) *Matrix Steps Dumbbell Flyes*
5 full reps
+
1 half-up
2 half-down
3 half-up
4 half-down
5 half-up
6 half-down
+
5 full reps

30 seconds pause

(f) *Iso-Matrix Steps Pec Deck*
     1 full rep
        +
     2 half-up (hold each rep for 3 seconds)
     3 half-down (hold each rep for 3 seconds)
     4 half-up (hold each rep for 3 seconds)
     5 half-down (hold each rep for 3 seconds)
        +
     6 full reps

     30 seconds pause

(g) *Matrix Composites Dumbbell Flyes*
     5 full reps
        +
     3 half-up
     3 half-down
        +
     3 half-up
     3 half-down
        +
     3 half-up
     3 half-down
        +
     5 full reps

     Finish

Thigh Matrix

Stage 4

Sequence A

(a) *Matrix Composites Leg Extensions*
     5 full reps
        +
     3 half-up
     3 half-down
        +
     3 half-up
     3 half-down
        +
     3 half-up
     3 half-down
        +
     5 full reps

     20 seconds pause

(b) *Matrix Reverse Step Ladders Leg Extensions*
     1 full rep
        +
     2 reps 1/5 up
     3 reps 1/5 down
        +
     4 reps 2/5 up
     5 reps 2/5 down
        +
     6 reps 3/5 up
     7 reps 3/5 down
        +
     8 reps 4/5 up
     9 reps 4/5 down
        +
     1 full rep

     25 seconds pause

(c) *Matrix Giant Steps Leg Extensions*
   5 full reps
      +
   1 half-up
   2 half-down
      +
   3 full reps
      +
   4 half-up
   5 half-down
      +
   6 full reps

   30 seconds pause

(d) *Matrix Reversals Leg Curls*
   5 full reps
      +
   1 rep 3/4 up
   1 rep 3/4 down
      +
   1 rep 3/4 up
   1 rep 3/4 down
      +
   1 rep 3/4 up
   1 rep 3/4 down
      +
   5 full reps

   30 seconds pause

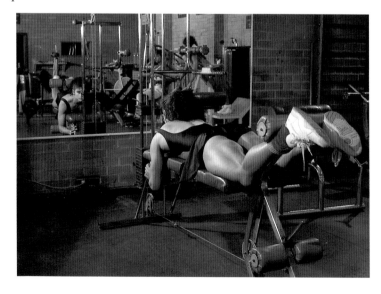

Matrix Reversals
Leg Curls

(e) *Matrix Reverse Ladders Leg Press*
5 full reps
+
1 rep 1/5 up
1 rep 1/5 down
+
1 rep 2/5 up
1 rep 2/5 down
+
1 rep 3/5 up
1 rep 3/5 down
+
1 rep 4/5 up
1 rep 4/5 down
+
5 full reps

35 seconds pause

(f) *Matrix Composites Leg Press*
5 full reps
+
3 half-up
3 half-down
+
3 half-up
3 half-down
+
3 half-up
3 half-down
+
5 full reps

35 seconds pause

(g) *Mixed iso-Matrix Leg Press*
5 full reps
+
3 half-up (hold each rep for 3 seconds)
3 half-down (no holding)
3 half-up (no holding)
3 half-down (hold each rep for 3 seconds)
+
5 full reps

3 minutes pause

Sequence B

(a) *Matrix Composites Squats*
   5 full reps
      +
   3 half-up
   3 half-down
      +
   3 half-up
   3 half-down
      +
   3 half-up
   3 half-down
      +
   5 full reps

   25 seconds pause

(b) *Matrix Reverse Ladders Squats*
   5 full reps
      +
   1 rep 1/5 up
   1 rep 1/5 down
      +
   1 rep 2/5 up
   1 rep 2/5 down
      +
   1 rep 3/5 up
   1 rep 3/5 down
      +
   1 rep 4/5 up
   1 rep 4/5 down
      +
   5 full reps

   45 seconds pause

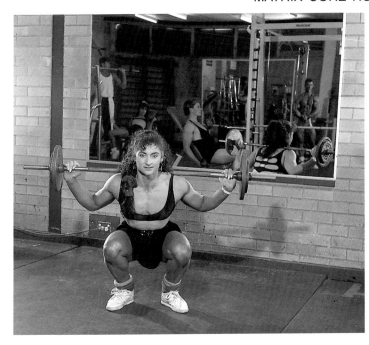

Matrix Giant
Steps Squats

(c) *Matrix Giant Steps Squats*
5 full reps
+
1 half-up
2 half-down
+
3 full reps
+
4 half-up
5 half-down
+
6 full reps

55 seconds pause

(d) *Iso-Matrix Steps Squats*
1 full rep
+
2 half-up (hold each rep for 3 seconds)
3 half-down (hold each rep for 3 seconds)
4 half-up (hold each rep for 3 seconds)
5 half-down (hold each rep for 3 seconds)
+
6 full reps

60 seconds pause

(e) *Cumulative Matrix Reversals Squats*
   3 full reps
      +
   3 reps 3/4 up
   3 reps 3/4 down
      +
   4 full reps
      +
   4 reps 3/4 up
   4 reps 3/4 down
      +
   5 full reps

   25 seconds pause

(f) *Matrix Composites Leg Curls*
   5 full reps
      +
   3 half-up
   3 half-down
      +
   3 half-up
   3 half-down
      +
   3 half-up
   3 half-down
      +
   5 full reps

   25 seconds pause

(g) *Matrix Reverse Step Ladders Leg Curls*
1 full rep
+
2 reps 1/5 up
3 reps 1/5 down
+
4 reps 2/5 up
5 reps 2/5 down
+
6 reps 3/5 up
7 reps 3/5 down
+
8 reps 4/5 up
9 reps 4/5 down
+
1 full rep

35 seconds pause

(h) *Iso-Matrix Giant Steps Leg Curls*
5 full reps
+
1 half-up (hold for 5 seconds)
2 half-down (hold each rep for 4 seconds)
+
3 full reps
+
4 half-up (hold each rep for 3 seconds)
5 half-down (hold each rep for 2 seconds)
+
6 full reps

40 seconds pause

(i) *Ascending Matrix Reversals Leg Curls*
5 full reps
+
1 rep 3/4 up
1 rep 3/4 down
+
6 full reps
+
1 rep 3/4 up
1 rep 3/4 down
+
7 full reps

Finish

Biceps Matrix

Stage 4

Sequence A

(a) *Matrix Composites Incline Bench Dumbbell Curls*
5 full reps
+
3 half-up
3 half-down
+
3 half-up
3 half-down
+
3 half-up
3 half-down
+
5 full reps

20 seconds pause

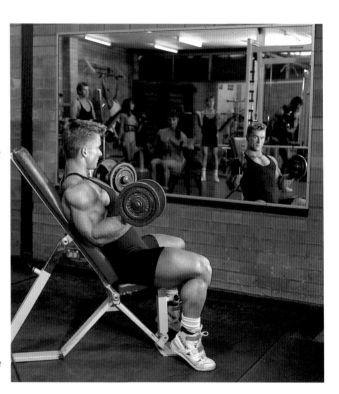

Matrix Composites Incline
Bench Dumbbell Curls

(b) *Cumulative Matrix Alternates Incline Bench Dumbbell Curls*

1 full rep	3 half-up
1 half-up	3 half-down
1 half-down	4 full reps
2 full reps +	+
+	4 half-up
2 half-up	4 half-down
2 half-down	5 full reps
3 full reps	

20 seconds pause

(c) *Matrix Reversals Incline Bench Dumbbell Curls*
  5 full reps
     +
  1 rep 3/4 up
  1 rep 3/4 down
     +
  1 rep 3/4 up
  1 rep 3/4 down
     +
  1 rep 3/4 up
  1 rep 3/4 down
     +
  5 full reps

  30 seconds pause

(d) *Iso-Matrix Steps Standing Barbell Curls*
  1 full rep
     +
  2 half-up (hold each rep for 3 seconds)
  3 half-down (hold each rep for 3 seconds)
  4 half-up (hold each rep for 3 seconds)
  5 half-down (hold each rep for 3 seconds)
     +
  6 full reps

  30 seconds pause

(e) *Mixed iso-Matrix Standing Barbell Curls*
  5 full reps
     +
  3 half-up (hold each rep for 3 seconds)
  3 half-down (no holding)
  3 half-up (no holding)
  3 half-down (hold each rep for 3 seconds)
     +
  5 full reps

  35 seconds pause

(f) *Matrix Giant Steps Barbell Curls*
     5 full reps
       +
     1 half-up
     2 half-down
       +
     3 full reps
       +
     4 half-up
     5 half-down
       +
     6 full reps

     40 seconds pause

(g) *Matrix Reverse Ladders Standing Barbell Curls*
     5 full reps
       +
     1 rep 1/5 up
     1 rep 1/5 down
       +
     1 rep 2/5 up
     1 rep 2/5 down
       +
     1 rep 3/5 up
     1 rep 3/5 down
       +
     1 rep 4/5 up
     1 rep 4/5 down
       +
     5 full reps

     3 minutes pause

Sequence B

(a) *Matrix Reverse Step Ladders Preacher Bench Curls*
   1 full rep
   +
   2 reps 1/5 up
   3 reps 1/5 down
   +
   4 reps 2/5 up
   5 reps 2/5 down
   +
   6 reps 3/5 up
   7 reps 3/5 down
   +
   8 reps 4/5 up
   9 reps 4/5 down
   +
   1 full rep

   25 seconds pause

(b) *Iso-Matrix Steps Preacher Bench Curls*
   1 full rep
   +
   2 half-up (hold each rep for 3 seconds)
   3 half-down (hold each rep for 3 seconds)
   4 half-up (hold each rep for 3 seconds)
   5 half-down (hold each rep for 3 seconds)
   +
   6 full reps

   30 seconds pause

(c) *Matrix Giant Steps Incline Bench Dumbbell Curls*
   5 full reps
   +
   1 half-up
   2 half-down
   +
   3 full reps
   +
   4 half-up
   5 half-down
   +
   6 full reps

   30 seconds pause

(d) *Matrix Steps Preacher Bench Curls*
   5 full reps
      +
   1 half-up
   2 half-down
   3 half-up
   4 half-down
   5 half-up
   6 half-down
      +
   5 full reps

   30 seconds pause

(e) *Cumulative iso-Matrix Barbell Curls*
   1 full rep
      +
   1 half-up (hold for 1 second)
   2 half-up (hold each rep for 2 seconds)
   3 half-up (hold each rep for 3 seconds)
   4 half-up (hold each rep for 4 seconds)
      +
   5 full reps
      +
   1 half-down (hold for 1 second)
   2 half-down (hold each rep for 2 seconds)
   3 half-down (hold each rep for 3 seconds)
   4 half-down (hold each rep for 4 seconds)
      +
   5 full reps

   Finish

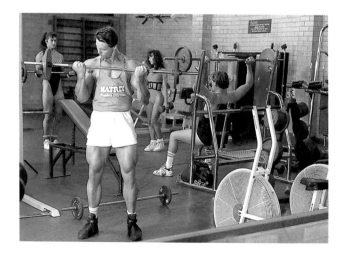

Cumulative iso-Matrix
Barbbell Curls

Triceps Matrix

Stage 4

Sequence A

(a) *Matrix Composites Lying Triceps Press*
   5 full reps
      +
   3 half-up
   3 half-down
      +
   3 half-up
   3 half-down
      +
   3 half-up
   3 half-down
      +
   5 full reps

   20 seconds pause

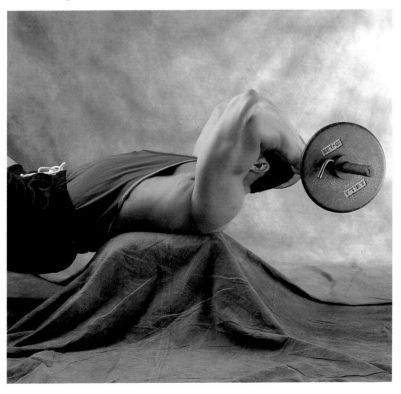

The finishing position of the Lying Triceps Press

(b) *Matrix Reverse Step Ladders Triceps Pushdowns*
1 full rep
+
2 reps 1/5 up
3 reps 1/5 down
+
4 reps 2/5 up
5 reps 2/5 down
+
6 reps 3/5 up
7 reps 3/5 down
+
8 reps 4/5 up
9 reps 4/5 down
+
1 full rep

25 seconds pause

(c) *Cumulative iso-Matrix Steps Triceps Pushdowns*
1 full rep
+
2 half-up (hold each rep for 3 seconds)
3 half-down (hold each rep for 4 seconds)
4 half-up (hold each rep for 5 seconds)
5 half-down (hold each rep for 6 seconds)
+
6 full reps

30 seconds pause

(d) *Matrix Giant Steps Triceps Pushdowns*
5 full reps
+
1 half-up
2 half-down
+
3 full reps
+
4 half-up
5 half-down
+
6 full reps

40 seconds pause

(e) *Matrix Reverse Ladders Standing Overhead Triceps Press*
5 full reps
+
1 rep 1/5 up
1 rep 1/5 down
+
1 rep 2/5 up
1 rep 2/5 down
+
1 rep 3/5 up
1 rep 3/5 down
+
1 rep 4/5 up
1 rep 4/5 down
+
5 full reps

40 seconds pause

(f) *Iso-Matrix Giant Steps Standing Overhead Triceps Press*
5 full reps
+
1 half-up (hold for 5 seconds)
2 half-down (hold each rep for 4 seconds)
+
3 full reps
+
4 half-up (hold each rep for 3 seconds)
5 half-down (hold each rep for 2 seconds)
+
6 full reps

40 seconds pause

(g) *Matrix Composites Standing Overhead Triceps Press*
5 full reps
+
3 half-up
3 half-down
+
3 half-up
3 half-down
+
3 half-up
3 half-down
+
5 full reps

30 seconds pause

(h) *Matrix Composites Triceps Pushdowns*
5 full reps
+
3 half-up
3 half-down
+
3 half-up
3 half-down
+
3 half-up
3 half-down
+
5 full reps

2 minutes pause

Sequence B

(a) *Matrix Reverse Ladders Lying Triceps Press*
    5 full reps
    +
    1 rep 1/5 up
    1 rep 1/5 down
    +
    1 rep 2/5 up
    1 rep 2/5 down
    +
    1 rep 3/5 up
    1 rep 3/5 down
    +
    1 rep 4/5 up
    1 rep 4/5 down
    +
    5 full reps

    25 seconds pause

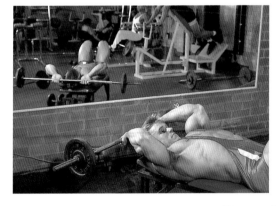

Lee Priest in the two-fifths from the bottom Matrix Ladder position.

(b) *Iso-Matrix Giant Steps Lying Triceps Press*
    5 full reps
    +
    1 half-up (hold for 5 seconds)
    2 half-down (hold each rep for 4 seconds)
    +
    3 full reps
    +
    4 half-up (hold each rep for 3 seconds)
    5 half-down (hold each rep for 2 seconds)
    +
    6 full reps

    25 seconds pause

(c) *Matrix Reversals Triceps Pushdowns*
5 full reps
+
1 rep 3/4 up
1 rep 3/4 down
+
1 rep 3/4 up
1 rep 3/4 down
+
1 rep 3/4 up
1 rep 3/4 down
+
5 full reps

30 seconds pause

(d) *Matrix Giant Steps Lying Triceps Press*
5 full reps
+
1 half-up
2 half-down
+
3 full reps
+
4 half-up
5 half-down
+
6 full reps

30 seconds pause

(e) *Matrix Composites Lying Triceps Press*
5 full reps
+
3 half-up
3 half-down
+
3 half-up
3 half-down
+
3 half-up
3 half-down
+
5 full reps

30 seconds pause

(f) *Cumulative iso-Matrix Steps Triceps Pushdowns*
     1 full rep
       +
     2 half-up (hold each rep for 3 seconds)
     3 half-down (hold each rep for 4 seconds)
     4 half-up (hold each rep for 5 seconds)
     5 half-down (hold each rep for 6 seconds)
       +
     6 full reps

     30 seconds pause

(g) *Matrix Steps Lying Triceps Press*
     5 full reps
       +
     1 half-up
     2 half-down
     3 half-up
     4 half-down
     5 half-up
     6 half-down
       +
     5 full reps

     Finish

Deltoid Matrix

Stage 4

Sequence A

(a) *Matrix Composites Dumbbell Lateral Raises*
     5 full reps
       +
     3 half-up
     3 half-down
       +
     3 half-up
     3 half-down
       +
     3 half-up
     3 half-down
       +
     5 full reps

     20 seconds pause

(b) *Matrix Reverse Ladders Dumbbell Lateral Raises*
   5 full reps
     +
   1 rep 1/5 up
   1 rep 1/5 down
     +
   1 rep 2/5 up
   1 rep 2/5 down
     +
   1 rep 3/5 up
   1 rep 3/5 down
     +
   1 rep 4/5 up
   1 rep 4/5 down
     +
   5 full reps

   25 seconds pause

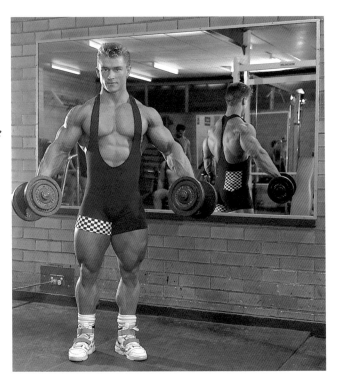

Matrix Reverse Ladders
Dumbbell Lateral Raises

(c) *Matrix Steps Dumbbell Front Raises*
   5 full reps
     +
   1 half-up
   2 half-down
   3 half-up
   4 half-down
   5 half-up
   6 half-down
     +
   5 full reps

   25 seconds pause

(d) *Cumulative Matrix Reversals Dumbbell Front Raises*
3 full reps
+
3 reps 3/4 up
3 reps 3/4 down
+
4 full reps
+
4 reps 3/4 up
4 reps 3/4 down
+
5 full reps

30 seconds pause

(e) *Matrix Roll Presses*
15 full reps
Note: The rest period between this set and the previous set may be adjusted to ensure that you can complete 15 reps.

30 seconds pause

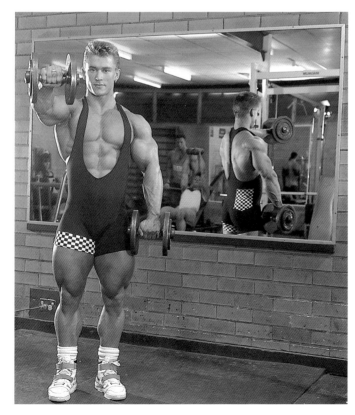

Cumulative Matrix
Reversals Dumbbell
Front Raises

(f) *Matrix Steps Roll Presses (as follows)*
5 full roll press reps
+
1 rep half-up in front of neck
+
1 roll press to the back of neck
+
2 reps half-up in back of neck
+
1 roll press to front of neck
+
3 reps half-up in front of neck
+
1 roll press to back of neck
+
4 reps half-up in back of neck
+
1 roll press to front of neck
+
5 reps half-up in front of neck
+
5 full roll press reps

30 seconds pause

(g) *Matrix Composites Roll Presses (as follows)*
5 full roll press reps
+
3 half-up in front of neck
+
3 half-down in front of neck
+
1 roll press to back of neck
+
3 half-up in back of neck
+
3 half-down in back of neck
+
5 full roll press reps

35 seconds pause

(h) *Matrix Reverse Ladders Press Behind the Neck*
5 full reps
   +
1 rep 1/5 up
1 rep 1/5 down
   +
1 rep 2/5 up
1 rep 2/5 down
   +
1 rep 3/5 up
1 rep 3/5 down
   +
1 rep 4/5 up
1 rep 4/5 down
   +
5 full reps

35 seconds pause

(i) *Iso-Matrix Giant Steps Press in Front of the Neck*
5 full reps
   +
1 half-up (hold for 5 seconds)
2 half-down (hold each rep for 4 seconds)
   +
3 full reps
   +
4 half-up (hold each rep for 3 seconds)
5 half-down (hold each rep for 2 seconds)
   +
6 full reps

35 seconds pause

(j) *Matrix Roll Presses*
15 reps or as many as possible up to 15

3 minutes pause

Sequence B

(a) *Matrix Composites Upright Rows*
   5 full reps
   +
   3 half-up
   3 half-down
   +
   3 half-up
   3 half-down
   +
   3 half-up
   3 half-down
   +
   5 full reps

   20 seconds pause

(b) *Matrix Reverse Step Ladders Behind the Neck*
   1 full rep
   +
   2 reps 1/5 up
   3 reps 1/5 down
   +
   4 reps 2/5 up
   5 reps 2/5 down
   +
   6 reps 3/5 up
   7 reps 3/5 down
   +
   8 reps 4/5 up
   9 reps 4/5 down
   +
   1 full rep

   25 seconds pause

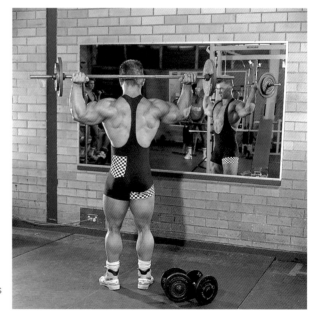

Matrix Reverse Step Ladders
Press Behind the Neck

(c) *Iso-Matrix Giant Steps Upright Rows*
5 full reps
\+
1 half-up (hold for 5 seconds)
2 half-down (hold each rep for 4 seconds)
\+
3 full reps
\+
4 half-up (hold each rep for 3 seconds)
5 half-down (hold each rep for 2 seconds)
\+
6 full reps

30 seconds pause

(d) *Cumulative Matrix Reversals Upright Rows*
3 full reps
\+
3 reps 3/4 up
3 reps 3/4 down
\+
4 full reps
\+
4 reps 3/4 up
4 reps 3/4 down
\+
5 full reps

30 seconds pause

(e) *Matrix Giant Steps Upright Rows*
5 full reps
\+
1 half-up
2 half-down
\+
3 full reps
\+
4 half-up
5 half-down
\+
6 full reps

Finish

Lats and Back Matrix

Stage 4

Sequence A

(a) *Matrix Composites Chin-Ups in Front of the Neck*
Modified as follows:
3 full reps
+
3 half-up
+
3 half-down
+
3 half-up
+
3 half-down
+
3 full reps

20 seconds pause

(b) *Matrix Composites Lat Machine Pulldowns*
5 full reps
+
3 half-up
3 half-down
+
3 half-up
3 half-down
+
3 half-up
3 half-down
+
5 full reps

25 seconds pause

(c) *Matrix Reverse Step Ladders Lat Machine Pulldowns*
1 full rep
+
2 reps 1/5 up
3 reps 1/5 down
+
4 reps 2/5 up
5 reps 2/5 down
+
6 reps 3/5 up
7 reps 3/5 down
+
8 reps 4/5 up
9 reps 4/5 down
+
1 full rep

30 seconds pause

(d) *Cumulative iso-Matrix Steps Lat Machine Pulldowns in Front of Neck*
1 full rep
+
2 half-up (hold each rep for 3 seconds)
3 half-down (hold each rep for 4 seconds)
4 half-up (hold each rep for 5 seconds)
5 half-down (hold each rep for 6 seconds)
+
6 full reps

35 seconds pause

(e) *Chin-Ups in Front of the Neck*
12 reps or as many as possible up to 12

35 seconds pause

(f) *Descending Matrix Reversals Lat Machine Pulldowns*
    7 full reps
    +
    1 rep 3/4 up
    1 rep 3/4 down
    +
    6 full reps
    +
    1 rep 3/4 up
    1 rep 3/4 down
    +
    5 full reps

    40 seconds pause

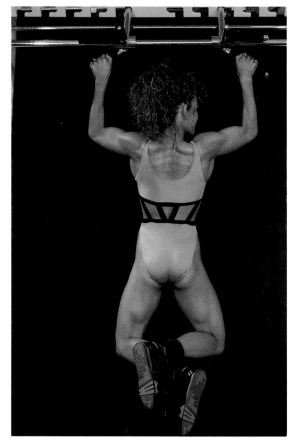

Gina Randall in the half-down
position of the iso-Matrix Steps
Chin-Ups.

(g) *Iso-Matrix Steps Chin-
    ups*
    1 full rep
    +
    2 half-up (hold each rep for 3 seconds)
    3 half-down (hold each rep for 3 seconds)
    4 half-up (hold each rep for 3 seconds)
    5 half-down (hold each rep for 3 seconds)
    +
    6 full reps

    40 seconds pause

(h) *Chin-Ups in Front of the Neck*
     12 reps or as many as possible up to 12

     3 minutes pause

Sequence B

(a) *Matrix Composites Bent-Over Rows*
     5 full reps
       +
     3 half-up
     3 half-down
       +
     3 half-up
     3 half-down
       +
     3 half-up
     3 half-down
       +
     5 full reps

     20 seconds pause

(b) *Matrix Reverse Step Ladders Bent-Over Rows*
     1 full rep
       +
     2 reps 1/5 up
     3 reps 1/5 down
       +
     4 reps 2/5 up
     5 reps 2/5 down
       +
     6 reps 3/5 up
     7 reps 3/5 down
       +
     8 reps 4/5 up
     9 reps 4/5 down
       +
     1 full rep

     25 seconds pause

(c) *Matrix Steps Hyperextensions*
5 full reps
+
1 half-up
2 half-down
3 half-up
4 half-down
5 half-up
6 half-down
+
5 full reps
25 seconds pause

(d) *Iso-Matrix Steps Hyperextensions*
1 full rep
+
2 half-up (hold each rep for 3 seconds)
3 half-down (hold each rep for 3 seconds)
4 half-up (hold each rep for 3 seconds)
5 half-down (hold each rep for 3 seconds)
+
6 full reps
30 seconds pause

(e) *Matrix Composites Hyperextensions*
5 full reps
+
3 half-up
3 half-down
+
3 half-up
3 half-down
+
3 half-up
3 half-down
+
5 full reps
30 seconds pause

(f) *Deadlifts*
12 reps or as many as possible up to 12
30 seconds pause

(g) *Bent-Arm Pullovers*
12 reps
30 seconds pause

(h) *Cumulative Matrix Reversals Bent-Over Rows*
3 full reps
+
3 reps 3/4 up
3 reps 3/4 down
+
4 full reps
+
4 reps 3/4 up
4 reps 3/4 down
+
5 full reps

35 seconds pause

(i) *Cumulative iso-Matrix Steps Bent-Over Rows*
1 full rep
+
2 half-up (hold each rep for 3 seconds)
3 half-down (hold each rep for 4 seconds)
4 half-up (hold each rep for 5 seconds)
5 half-down (hold each rep for 6 seconds)
+
6 full reps

30 seconds pause

(j) *Bent-Arm Pullovers*
12 reps

30 seconds pause

(k) *Matrix Giant Steps Bent-Over Rows*
5 full reps
+
1 half-up
2 half-down
+
3 full reps
+
4 half-up
5 half-down
+
6 full reps

Finish

6   Matrix specialisation routines

Specialisation routines are provided here for the three main body parts not covered in the core routines (see p.27): the abdominals, calves and forearms. Many weight trainers who have a good overall development nonetheless find that they have a weakness in one or more of these 'problem' areas, resulting in an imbalance in the physique. Others, perhaps because of genetic factors, are lucky enough not to have to spend a lot of time on these body parts: they seem to be blessed by nature with washboard abs, diamond calves or full, rounded forearm flexors. Most, however, are not so lucky.

If you have a weakness in one, two or all of these areas, you should not give up trying but rather pay special attention to the problem body part or parts. Even Arnold Schwarzenegger, in his early bodybuilding days, had great difficulty in building up his calves to the same level of development as the rest of his body. The success of his 'blitzing' campaign, and the impressive calf development that resulted, are a reminder that perseverance and concentrated attention can overcome the challenge presented by even the most stubborn body part.

The specialisation routines, then, will be used by different trainers to different degrees, depending on the extent to which they need to devote special attention to one or more of these problem areas. In that sense, they differ from the standard programme which is the same for all trainers. You can therefore adapt your weekly training schedule by using the available time-slots to work hard on any areas of weakness.

The routines set out below are each divided into three sequences (A, B and C), all of which should be performed in a single workout session. You will note that the exercises are of two kinds: Matrix and 'standard' exercises. As with the other exercises in this book, those exercises which are not described as 'Matrix' are all meant to be performed as normal or standard weight-training exercises for the number of repetitions given.

The Matrix exercises shown in this section are all set out as 'conventional' Matrix; that is to be performed according to the simplest of the Matrix techniques (5 full, 5 half-up, 5 half-down, 5 full). To get the most out of

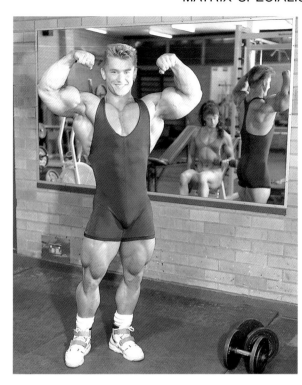

Lee Priest displays his overall
massive muscle development.

the specialisation routines, however, you would do well to replace the
conventional Matrix movements with progressively more difficult Matrix
sequences as your ability improves. Following this programme, you will
thus perform the routine as set out for the *first two weeks* only; for the next
two weeks, you will replace the conventional Matrix movements by descending Matrix; for the following two weeks, you will replace the descending
Matrix movements by ascending Matrix; and so on. In accordance with this
schedule, you will perform the Matrix movements as set out in the table
which follows.

Weeks 1 and 2	Conventional Matrix
Weeks 3 and 4	Descending Matrix
Weeks 5 and 6	Ascending Matrix
Weeks 7 and 8	Matrix Alternates
Weeks 9 and 10	Cumulative Matrix Alternates
Weeks 11 and 12	Matrix Ladders
Weeks 13 and 14	Cumulative Matrix Ladders

Weeks 15 and 16	Ascending Iso-Matrix
Weeks 17 and 18	Descending Iso-Matrix
Weeks 19 and 20	Conventional Iso-Matrix
Weeks 21 and 22	Cumulative Iso-Matrix
Weeks 23 and 24	Mixed Iso-Matrix
Weeks 25 and 26	Matrix Steps
Weeks 27 and 28	Matrix Giant Steps
Weeks 29 and 30	Iso-Matrix Steps
Weeks 31 and 32	Cumulative Iso-Matrix Steps
Weeks 33 and 34	Iso-Matrix Giant Steps
Weeks 35 and 36	Matrix Reversals
Weeks 37 and 38	Descending Matrix Reversals
Weeks 39 and 40	Ascending Matrix Reversals
Weeks 41 and 42	Cumulative Matrix Reversals
Weeks 43 and 44	Matrix Composites
Weeks 45 and 46	Matrix Reverse Ladders
Weeks 47 and 48	Matrix Reverse Step Ladders

Abdominal specialisation

Sequence A

(a) *Conventional Matrix Incline Board Sit-Ups*
    5 full reps
    5 half-up
    5 half-down
    5 full reps

    30 seconds pause

(b) *Incline Board Leg Raises*
    15 full reps

    30 seconds pause

(c) *Conventional Matrix Hanging Leg Raises*
5 full reps
5 half-up
5 half-down
5 full reps

3 minutes pause

Sequence B

(a) *Conventional Matrix Incline Board Leg Raises*
5 full reps
5 half-up
5 half-down
5 full reps

30 seconds pause

(b) *Hanging Leg Raises*
12 full reps

30 seconds pause

(c) *Conventional Matrix Incline Board Sit-Ups*
5 full reps
5 half-up
5 half-down
5 full reps

3 minutes pause

Sequence C

(a) *Conventional Matrix Hanging Leg Raises*
5 full reps
5 half-up
5 half-down
5 full reps

30 seconds pause

(b) *Incline Board Sit-Ups*
12-15 full reps

30 seconds pause

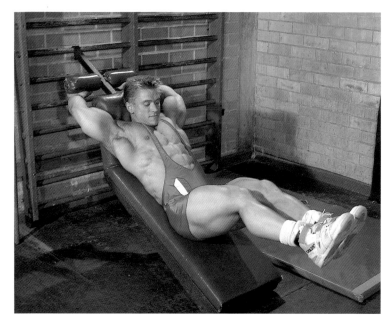

Conventional Matrix Incline Board Leg Raises

(c) *Conventional Matrix Incline Board Leg Raises*
   5 full reps
   5 half-up
   5 half-down
   5 full reps

   Finish

Calf specialisation

Sequence A

(a) *Standing Calf Raises (warm-up)*
   15 full reps (hold 1 second at top and bottom of movement)

   20 seconds pause

Sequence B

(b) *Conventional Matrix Standing Calf Raises*
   5 full reps
   5 half-up
   5 half-down
   5 full reps

   15 seconds pause

(c) *Conventional Matrix Seated Calf Raises*
     5 full reps
     5 half-up
     5 half-down
     5 full reps

     1 minute pause

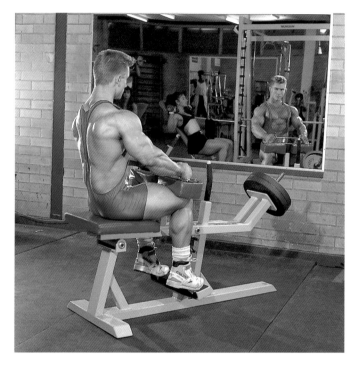

Conventional Matrix
Donkey Calf Raises

Sequence C

(d) *Conventional Matrix Donkey Calf Raises*
     5 full reps
     5 half-up
     5 half-down
     5 full reps

     1 minute pause

(e) *Conventional Matrix Standing Calf Raises*
     5 full reps (hold 2 seconds at top and bottom of movement)
     5 half-up (hold 1 second)
     5 half-down
     5 full reps (no holding)

     Finish

Forearm specialisation

Sequence A

(a) *Conventional Matrix Reverse Wrist Curls*
    5 full reps
    5 half-up
    5 half-down
    5 full reps

    20 seconds pause

(b) *Conventional Matrix Wrist Curls*
    5 full reps
    5 half-up
    5 half-down
    5 full reps

    30 seconds pause

(c) *Conventional Matrix Reverse Wrist Curls*
    5 full reps
    5 half-up
    5 half-down
    5 full reps

    1 minute pause

Sequence B

(a) *Conventional Matrix Reverse Wrist Curls*
    5 full reps
    5 half-up
    5 half-down
    5 full reps

    30 seconds pause

(b) *Reverse Wrist Curls*
    15-20 reps

    50 seconds pause

(c) *Conventional Matrix Wrist Curls*
    5 full reps
    5 half-up
    5 half-down
    5 full reps

    3 minutes pause

Sequence C

(a) *Conventional Matrix Wrist Curls*
5 full reps
5 half-up
5 half-down
5 full reps

30 seconds pause

(b) *Forearm Curls*
12-15 reps

50 seconds pause

(c) *Conventional Matrix Reverse Wrist Curls*
5 full reps
5 half-up
5 half-down
5 full reps

60 seconds pause

(d) *Reverse Forearm Curls*
15 reps

60 seconds pause

(e) *Conventional Matrix Reverse Wrist Curls*
5 full reps
5 half-up
5 half-down
5 full reps

Finish

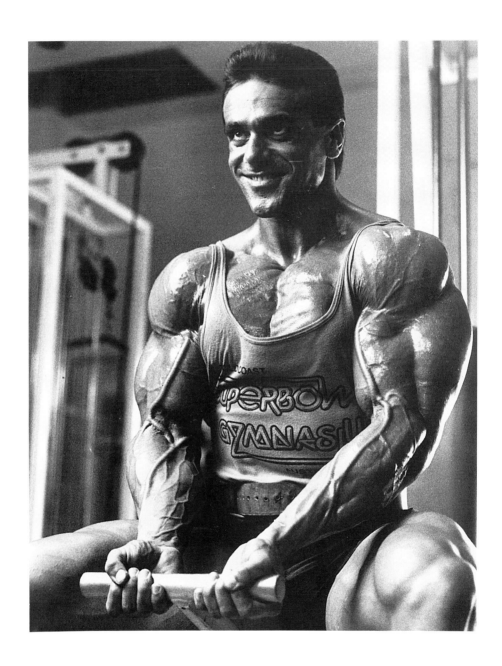

THE MATRIX PRINCIPLE

By Ronald S. Laura and Kenneth R. Dutton

The Matrix Principle introduces the MATRIX System, a major breakthrough in weight training for all those seeking to build a healthy and muscular physique **without the use of harmful drugs**.

Using clear and comprehensive instructions, *The Matrix Principle* provides a complete set of workout routines for each body part. It introduces trainers to the most effective methods of aerobic, isometric and isotonic weight training as well as the most recent advances in exercise physiology, explaining how and why muscles grow and why some forms of exercise are more effective than others in fostering muscle development.

The Matrix Principle is for trainers at all levels from amateur and professional sports people and contest winning bodybuilders to those just wanting to improve their general fitness.

TWELVE WEEKS TO A BETTER BODY FOR WOMEN
TWELVE WEEKS TO A BETTER BODY FOR MEN

Two new books by Ronald S. Laura and Kenneth R. Dutton

These two compact books show how a revolutionary form of light-weight exercise can be used to tone up the most out-of-shape body.

The revolutionary MATRIX System, which has proved itself several times more effective than conventional exercise methods, has now been adapted to meet the needs of men and women who have never exercised before or who have let themselves get out of condition. The daily exercise programmes require no special equipment and are easy to follow and simple to perform. Helpful dietary advice is also provided.